IPCS

INTERNATIONAL PROGRAMME ON CHEMICAL SAFETY

Environmental Health Criteria 243

AIRCRAFT DISINSECTION INSECTICIDES

IOMC

INTER-ORGANIZATION PROGRAMME FOR THE SOUND MANAGEMENT OF CHEMICALS

A cooperative agreement among FAO, ILO, UNDP, UNEP, UNIDO, UNITAR, WHO, World Bank and OECD

This report contains the collective views of an international group of experts and does not necessarily represent the decisions or the stated policy of the World Health Organization

World Health Organization

The **International Programme on Chemical Safety (IPCS)** was established in 1980. The overall objectives of the IPCS are to establish the scientific basis for assessment of the risk to human health and the environment from exposure to chemicals, through international peer review processes, as a prerequisite for the promotion of chemical safety, and to provide technical assistance in strengthening national capacities for the sound management of chemicals.

This publication was developed in the IOMC context. The contents do not necessarily reflect the views or stated policies of individual IOMC Participating Organizations.

The **Inter-Organization Programme for the Sound Management of Chemicals (IOMC)** was established in 1995 following recommendations made by the 1992 UN Conference on Environment and Development to strengthen cooperation and increase international coordination in the field of chemical safety. The Participating Organizations are: FAO, ILO, UNDP, UNEP, UNIDO, UNITAR, WHO, World Bank and OECD. The purpose of the IOMC is to promote coordination of the policies and activities pursued by the Participating Organizations, jointly or separately, to achieve the sound management of chemicals in relation to human health and the environment.

WHO Library Cataloguing-in-Publication Data

Aircraft disinsection insecticides.

(Environmental health criteria; 243)

1. Insect control. 2. Disinfection – methods. 3. Aircraft. 4. Aerospace medicine. 5. Insecticides. I. World Health Organization.

ISBN 978 92 4 157243 9 (NLM classification: WD 700)
ISSN 0250-863X

The preparation of this report was funded by the European Commission and the Policy Research Programme of the United Kingdom Department of Health. The views expressed in this report do not necessarily reflect the views of these two organizations.

CONTENTS

TERMINOLOGY, ABBREVIATIONS AND ACRONYMS

ADI	acceptable daily intake
a.i.	active ingredient
AOEL	acceptable operator exposure level
ARfD	acute reference dose
ATSDR	Agency for Toxic Substances and Disease Registry
BMD	benchmark dose
BMDL	lower 95% confidence limit on the BMD
EFSA	European Food Safety Authority
GLP	good laboratory practice
guideline scenario	the insecticide is used according to the instructions given on the product label and in WHO guideline information
IARC	International Agency for Research on Cancer
IHR	International Health Regulations (2005)
IPCS	International Programme on Chemical Safety
JECFA	Joint FAO/WHO Expert Committee on Food Additives
JMPM	Joint FAO/WHO Meeting on Pesticide Management
JMPR	Joint FAO/WHO Meeting on Pesticide Residues
lax standard scenario	a scenario representing less than optimum conditions, such as minor deviations from instructions, missing or inadequate protective clothing, equipment not functioning perfectly
LD_{50}	median lethal dose
LOAEL	lowest-observed-adverse-effect level
NOAEC	no-observed-adverse-effect concentration
NOAEL	no-observed-adverse-effect level
OECD	Organisation for Economic Co-operation and Development
OEL	occupational exposure level
PPE	personal protective equipment

PSD	Pesticides Safety Directorate of the United Kingdom
RfC	reference concentration
RfD	reference dose
TSD	tolerable systemic dose
TSD_{AC}	tolerable systemic dose for acute exposure
TWA	time-weighted average
UF	uncertainty factor
USEPA	United States Environmental Protection Agency
WHO	World Health Organization

PREFACE

The Environmental Health Criteria monographs are intended to assist national and international authorities in making risk assessments and subsequent risk management decisions. They represent a thorough evaluation of risks and are not, in any sense, recommendations for regulation or standard setting. These latter are the exclusive purview of national and regional governments.

The World Health Organization, through the International Health Regulations (2005), recommends the use of disinsection techniques in aircraft to help to minimize the spread of mosquito-borne diseases. The control measures recommended by WHO include the use of chemical insecticides (WHO, 1985). WHO has published generic human health risk assessment models for insecticides used for other public health purposes (WHO, 2011a and 2011b), and a decision was taken by WHO to develop a risk assessment model for aircraft disinsection insecticides, based on the same principles. In order to assist Member States who are required to assess aircraft disinsection insecticides within their jurisdiction, a number of product types currently used or proposed for use have been evaluated according to the risk assessment model.

In this publication, the generic risk assessment model (with worked examples) is presented first, in Part A, along with the description of the process used to develop the model. The evaluation of the different types of aircraft disinsection product against the risk assessment model is presented in Part B.

PART A

A GENERIC RISK ASSESSMENT MODEL FOR DISINSECTION OF AIRCRAFT WITH CHEMICAL INSECTICIDES

ACKNOWLEDGEMENTS

The first draft of this generic model was prepared at the request of the World Health Organization by the Finnish Institute of Occupational Health, Kuopio, Finland. The work was led by M. Koponen. The first draft was subject to a public review period and comments were received from the following individuals and organizations: A. Aitio, Finland; A. Evans, International Civil Aviation Organization, Montreal, Canada; D. Farr, Ministry for Primary Industries, Auckland, New Zealand; A. Grimes, Callington Haven Pty Ltd, Rydalmere, Australia; R. Kleinpaste, Auckland, New Zealand; J. Leung, Pest Management Regulatory Agency, Ottawa, Canada; T. Phelan, Department of Health and Ageing, Canberra, Australia; J. Sventek, Aerospace Medical Association, Alexandria, VA, USA; C. Thibeault, International Air Transport Association, Montreal, Canada; C. Tomicic, Federal Office of Public Health, Bern, Switzerland; E. Trajber, Produits Sanitaires Aéronefs, Croissy Beaubourg, France; and J. van Engelen, National Institute for Public Health and the Environment (RIVM), Bilthoven, Netherlands. Technical advice was also provided by Airbus.

The comments received were considered by the Secretariat with the assistance of M. Koponen. A revised draft of the document was then reviewed and presented at a WHO Expert Consultation held at Imperial College London, England, on 11–12 January 2012. The experts appointed by WHO were A. Aitio, Finland; S. Batt, Department of Health and Ageing, Canberra, Australia; A. Boobis, Imperial College London, England; D. Farr, Ministry for Primary Industries, Auckland, New Zealand; M. Koponen, Finnish Institute of Occupational Health, Kuopio, Finland; N. Morgan, Chemicals Regulatory Directorate, York, England; and J. van Engelen, National Institute for Public Health and the Environment (RIVM), Bilthoven, Netherlands. None of the participating experts declared an interest related to the subject matter of this consultation which could have given rise to a conflict. The Secretariat was provided by WHO, assisted by P. Howe, Peterborough, England.

The WHO Expert Consultation was preceded by a Stakeholder Workshop held on 10 January 2012 at Imperial College London, England, in the presence of the WHO-appointed experts, for the purposes of providing information and the exchange of views. The

Stakeholder Workshop was open to all interested parties. To this end, announcements for the Stakeholder Workshop were sent to a wide range of umbrella organizations and professional associations who represented stakeholders from different sectors (e.g. insecticide manufacturers, airlines, aviation medicine associations, trade unions in the transport sector) plus a number of government departments with an interest in aircraft disinsection. Representatives from the following organizations participated (either in person or making presentations via webinar): Produits Sanitaires Aéronefs; LKC Switzerland Ltd; Sumi Agro France, Sumitomo Corporation Group; Callington Haven Pty Ltd; US Department of Transportation; International Civil Aviation Organization; International Air Transport Association; Association of Flight Attendants/International Transport Workers Federation.

After being finalized by the WHO-appointed experts, the document was prepared for editing by the WHO Secretariat assisted by P. Howe. The document was edited by S. Ballance.

R. Brown, Department of Public Health and Environment, WHO, Geneva, Switzerland, served as the Responsible Officer for this publication in WHO.

The preparation of this report was funded by the European Commission and the Policy Research Programme of the United Kingdom Department of Health. The views expressed in this report do not necessarily reflect the views of these two organizations.

The assistance of the individuals and organizations listed above is gratefully acknowledged.

1. INTRODUCTION

WHO defines "disinsection" as the procedure whereby health measures are taken to control or kill the insect vectors of human diseases present in baggage, cargo, containers, conveyances, goods and postal parcels. Long-standing WHO recommendations cover the use of disinsection techniques in aircraft to help to minimize the spread of mosquito-borne diseases (WHO, 1985). Mosquitoes act as vectors of pathogens and parasites that cause a number of serious diseases, including dengue, yellow fever and malaria (WHO, 2005a). The *International Health Regulations (2005)* (IHR) establish global benchmark standards to prevent, protect against, control and provide a public health response to the international spread of disease in ways that are commensurate with and restricted to public health risks and that avoid unnecessary interference with international traffic and trade (WHO, 2005a). Control measures for the disinsection of aircraft are referred to in Annex 5 of the IHR, "Specific measures for vector-borne diseases", which states (clause 2) that, where there are methods and materials advised by WHO for disinsection, these should be employed and that (clause 3) States should accept disinsection if methods and materials advised by WHO have been employed.

Residual disinsection provides an insecticidal deposit on inside walls of structures (cargo areas or passenger cabins) to kill target insects that come into contact with the treated surface. Such deposits are intended to remain active for extended periods of time.

Space spraying is the dissemination of small particles (under 30 μm) that will remain airborne sufficiently long (usually not more than 30 minutes) to make contact with flying target species. This type of treatment involves a very low dosage of insecticide as it is not intended to leave a residual deposit.

For aircraft disinsection, WHO currently recommends *d*-phenothrin (2%) for space spraying and permethrin (2%) for residual disinsection (WHO, 2005b).

The WHO recommendations for methods and insecticides to be used for aircraft disinsection were considered in 1995 during an Informal Consultation that described methods, specifications for aerosols and solvents, and recommended insecticides to be used with particular methods (WHO, 1995). The toxicity of the pyrethroid insecticides recommended by WHO for aircraft disinsection was reviewed (along with other public health uses) in 2005 (WHO, 2005b). The following recommended methods were included in these publications:

- Pre-flight spraying, which involves the aircraft cabin being sprayed with an aerosol containing a residual insecticide while the aircraft is on the ground but before passengers embark. Pre-flight spraying may be combined with blocks-away or top-of-descent spraying.
- Residual spraying, which involves the regular application of a residual insecticide to internal surfaces of the aircraft, except in food preparation areas, at intervals based on the duration of effectiveness. In addition, spot applications are made to surfaces that are frequently cleaned.
- Blocks-away spraying, which involves aerosol spraying of the passenger cabin after the doors have been locked following embarkation but before take-off.
- Top-of-descent spraying, which is in-flight spraying carried out as the aircraft starts its descent to the destination airport.

The WHO recommendations published to date have covered both the efficacy and human health aspects of aircraft disinsection products (based on published studies).

Reports completed by flight attendants or airline personnel have suggested the possibility of the onset of symptoms in passengers and crew members as a consequence of pyrethroid application. The reported symptoms varied from metallic taste, slight and nonspecific irritation of eyes, throat and upper respiratory tract and, in some cases, skin, to severe respiratory symptoms such as dyspnoea, cough and even asthma. In other cases headache and allergic reactions were reported.

According to a WHO report (WHO, 2005b), available data suggest that the most severe symptoms were observed in sensitized subjects (i.e. asthma patients) and were attributed by the affected subjects to aircraft disinsection. However, WHO points out that many of the reports lack details, such as the type of active ingredient or the application method used; moreover, the symptoms observed in most of the reported cases are not typical of those from pyrethroids and might be attributable to other etiological factors.

To date, no widely-accepted, peer-reviewed human health risk assessment model for aircraft disinsection insecticides has been available. This document now describes a generic human health risk assessment model that can be used to evaluate both existing and proposed new insecticide products for aircraft disinsection (by residual treatment and space spraying, including new methods not previously recommended). It has the potential to harmonize the procedures that may be used by national regulatory authorities when registering these products. Nevertheless, the requirements for registration of pesticides are determined by the national regulatory authorities.

This document was developed by a process incorporating review by individuals and institutions known for their expertise in the subject. Following public and peer review, a revised draft was discussed at an Expert Consultation convened by WHO at Imperial College, London, England, on 11–12 January 2012, where WHO-appointed experts finalized the document by consensus. The Expert Consultation was preceded by a Stakeholder Workshop on 10 January 2012, open to all interested parties, which was attended by representatives of pesticides manufacturers, cabin crew organizations and international aviation organizations, alongside the WHO-appointed experts, for the purpose of exchanging information and views.

The scope of this document is restricted to human health risk assessment: the efficacy of products and the circumstances in which aircraft disinsection should be undertaken are not considered. Guidance on testing the efficacy of insecticide products used in aircraft has been published separately (WHO, 2012a).

2. PURPOSE

This document provides a generic model that can be used for risk assessment of exposure to insecticide products applied for aircraft disinsection. WHO-recommended residual disinsection performed as a ground procedure and space spraying during flight have been used as example procedures. Since other possible treatment methods are similar to the two that are described in detail, the same models can be used to estimate the risk in other scenarios, with only small modifications of default values, etc. It should be noted that relatively non-volatile insecticides applied with hydraulic spray equipment or via aerosol cans have been assumed for this model.

The document aims to harmonize the risk assessment of such insecticides in order to generate comparable data for registering and labelling of products by national regulatory authorities. The assessment considers:

- those applying (and, when necessary, preparing) the spray, i.e. ground service staff or cabin crew;
- passengers of the treated aircraft (adults, children, toddlers and newborn infants).

Both direct and indirect exposures of the groups listed above from both residual and space spraying have been assessed. The disinsection procedures and related exposures are fully outlined in this document, the structure of which follows that of other published risk assessment documents for insecticides used for public health purposes – for example, *A generic risk assessment model for insecticide-treated nets* (WHO, 2012b). Because risk assessment is a constantly evolving process and guidance must necessarily be subject to change, readers are advised to consider any more recent guidance published by WHO and other authoritative sources.

Issues related to insecticides for indoor residual spraying, including criteria for substance selection, are broadly discussed in a WHO publication of 2001 (Najera & Zaim, 2001); for space spraying in public health, the procedures and equipment for application are detailed in a practitioner's guide (WHO, 2003).

Generic risk assessment models for indoor residual and space spraying of insecticides for public health purposes in dwellings and residential areas have also been published by WHO (WHO, 2011a and 2011b), and many of the same principles are followed in this document.

The purpose of this document is to assist governmental organizations in WHO Member States in decision-making when considering aircraft disinsection within their jurisdiction. It should be noted, however, that the regulatory approval of products and methods for aircraft disinsection is the sole prerogative and responsibility of national authorities.

3. BACKGROUND

It is recommended that the risk assessments for insecticides proposed for aircraft disinsection are not conducted de novo; risk assessments that have already been undertaken for the pesticides in the regulatory context of crop protection can be used as a starting point. Preference should be for international assessments, followed by peer-reviewed regional or national assessments; risk assessments published in reputable journals would be a third possible source.

For each component of the risk assessment, any additional information – or modification of the existing assessment – likely to be needed will be identified and discussed. It is assumed that the generic guidance given here will be followed in parallel with one of the published regulatory schemes. These regulatory schemes are intended for guidance and none is wholly prescriptive; all state specifically that expert judgement is required.

Historically, exposure models have been based on point estimates. This deterministic approach, as applied in this document, has the advantage of simplicity and consistency. Moreover, risk characterization is quite straightforward, involving comparison of exposure estimate with a health-based guidance value. The drawback of the deterministic approach is that it does not incorporate information about the variability of real exposures, nor is the uncertainty in the exposure estimate assessed or communicated.

WHO encourages everyone using the models published here to consider probabilistic exposure assessment as an alternative, especially when higher-tier assessments are necessary. Such probabilistic models may provide alternative ways of establishing acceptable exposure levels in the future (WHO, 2009).

3.1 Description of aircraft disinsection procedures

The disinsection procedures that are described here mostly follow WHO's *Report of the Informal Consultation on Aircraft Disinsection* (WHO, 1995). The Schedule of Aircraft Disinsection Procedures developed by the governments of Australia and New Zealand

(DAFF/MPI, 2012) is also used as a source of information. These two documents give more detailed descriptions of the actual procedures.

3.1.1 Residual disinsection

The residual disinsection method involves the regular spraying of certain internal surfaces of the aircraft cabin (excluding food preparation areas) and hold with a residual insecticide; this ensures that, if an insect gains access to the aircraft and lands on a surface, it will receive an effective dose of insecticide. Treatment must be repeated at intervals not exceeding eight weeks. Any treated areas subsequently deep cleaned or refurbished within the treatment interval must be retreated to ensure compliance (WHO, 1995).

3.1.2 Pre-embarkation cabin disinsection

The pre-embarkation cabin disinsection system was developed in Australia and New Zealand and provides for the spraying of aircraft cabins in the absence of passengers, i.e. before embarkation. The treatment lasts for the duration of the single flight sector. This method not only kills invertebrates that may be present in the cabin at the time of disinsection but also leaves a minimal but effective amount of residue which is likely to kill invertebrates that may board between the time of disinsection and departure. The number of insects that enter a treated cabin between these times may be fewer than enter an untreated cabin because of the repellent effect of permethrin (WHO, 1995; R. Kleinpaste, personal communication).

Spraying is carried out using 2% permethrin aerosols. All overhead lockers are opened, and the cockpit, toilets, wardrobes and other insect harbourage areas such as the galley are also treated at this time. This treatment is carried out in conjunction with a suitable hold treatment option (residual or aerosol).

3.1.3 Blocks away disinsection

"Blocks away" disinsection takes place before take-off but after passengers have boarded and the doors have been closed. The aircraft is treated by cabin crew members walking through the cabins discharging aerosols at the prescribed dosage (spray cans). Crew must treat all possible insect harbourages, including toilets, galleys, wardrobes and lockers. Holds and the flight deck are sprayed before departure – the flight deck before boarding by the crew.

3.1.4 Pre-flight and top-of-descent spraying

Pre-flight and top-of-descent spraying is a two-part process. The pre-flight spray is carried out before the passengers board and is usually performed in conjunction with a pre-flight disinsection of the hold. The timing of this spray allows lockers to be open and causes minimum inconvenience to passengers. A subsequent in-flight spraying is carried out at "top-of-descent", i.e. as the aircraft starts its descent to the destination airport.

3.2 Essential elements of a risk assessment model

Comprehensive presentations on the principles of risk assessment can be found elsewhere in the scientific literature (e.g. WHO, 1999; WHO, 2009); only a short summary is given here.

Hazard is defined as the inherent capacity of a chemical substance to cause adverse effects in humans, other animals and/or the environment. *Risk* is defined as the probability that a particular adverse effect will be observed under certain conditions of *exposure* or use. *Risk characterization* is the process of combining hazard and exposure information to describe the likelihood of occurrence and the severity of adverse effects associated with a particular exposure in a given population. The entire process of hazard assessment, exposure estimation and risk characterization is known as *risk assessment*. Identification and expression of the *uncertainties* related to all aspects of a risk assessment are essential parts of a valid, good-quality risk assessment.

The subsequent process of *risk management* considers the risk assessment and attendant uncertainties in parallel with any potential benefits, socioeconomic and political factors, the possibilities for risk reduction and other issues that are relevant in making operational decisions on the acceptability of a particular level of risk.

Risk assessments involve three steps:

- ***Hazard assessment.*** Hazard assessment comprises hazard identification and hazard characterization, i.e. identification of the possible toxic effects of a substance, the dose/exposure levels at which those effects occur, and the dose/exposure levels below which no adverse effects are observed.
- ***Exposure assessment.*** Exposure assessment may concern those applying pesticides (usually referred to as operators or applicators) and those others who are either present when pesticides are applied or subsequently come into contact with treated areas. All exposure scenarios must be considered. Exposure should be assessed in a "*guideline scenario*", which assumes that the insecticide is used according to the instructions given on the product label and in WHO guideline information. In reality, however, these instructions may not be followed completely (or equipment may not function perfectly), and exposure should therefore also be assessed in what is termed a "*lax standard scenario*". Conservative, high-end point estimates of the default distributions are used as defaults. Intentional misuse is not considered. All relevant routes of exposure – oral, dermal and inhalational – are covered.
- ***Risk characterization.*** In the risk characterization step, estimates of exposure are compared with acceptable exposure levels previously established in hazard assessment in all relevant exposure situations and subpopulations.

The various sections of this document deal with specific information demands, data sources, uncertainties, vulnerable or sensitive subgroups, selection of default values and the underlying assumptions, etc.

4. THE HUMAN HEALTH RISK ASSESSMENT MODEL

4.1 Hazard assessment (hazard identification and hazard characterization)

The purpose of human health hazard assessment is to identify:

- whether an agent may pose a health hazard to human health; and
- the circumstances in which the hazard may be expressed (WHO, 1999; WHO, 2009).

It involves the weight-of-evidence assessment of all available data on toxicity, mode of action and all other relevant information such as physicochemical properties, metabolic fate and the establishment of dose–response curves and the threshold level below which the effects are no longer observed. The principles of human health hazard assessment are discussed in greater detail elsewhere (e.g. WHO, 1999; WHO, 2009); they are largely the same, regardless of the class of chemical or its use pattern, and differ only in, for example, data requirements. These principles have also been summarized in an earlier WHO publication (WHO, 2011), which describes a generic risk assessment model for insecticide treatment and subsequent use of mosquito nets and which, with some updating, is used as a basis for the current text.

4.1.1 Sources of data

Hazard identification is based on gathering and analysing relevant data on the possible effects of the insecticide on humans. These data may include both toxicological (animal testing) and human data. It is recommended that, when available, authoritative risk assessments that have already been generated for the insecticides, e.g. in the regulatory context of crop protection, be used as a starting point. These risk assessments usually contain all the relevant health hazard data available for the insecticide in question and are therefore important sources of information. Preference should be for international assessments, followed by peer-reviewed regional or national assessments; evaluations published in reputable, peer-reviewed journals are also possible sources.

Table 1. Examples of authoritative evaluations that may be used as a starting point for the risk assessment of aircraft disinsection insecticides

Joint Meeting on Pesticide Residues (JMPR) – Monographs and Evaluations	http://www.inchem.org/pages/jmpr.html
Joint Expert Committee on Food Additives (JECFA)	http://www.inchem.org/pages/jecfa.html
International Programme on Chemical Safety (IPCS)	http://www.inchem.org/pages/cicads.html
– Concise International Chemical Assessment Documents	http://www.inchem.org/pages/ehc.html
– Environmental Health Criteria Monographs	
International Agency for Research on Cancer (IARC) – Monographs on the Evaluation of Carcinogenic Risks to Humans	http://monographs.iarc.fr/
US Environmental Protection Agency (USEPA) – Pesticide evaluations	http://www.epa.gov/pesticides/regulating/index.htm, or http://www.epa.gov/pesticides/reregistration/status.htm
Agency for Toxic Substances and Disease Registry (ATSDR) – Toxicological Profiles	http://www.atsdr.cdc.gov/toxpro2.html
European Food Safety Authority (EFSA) – Pesticide Risk Assessments	http://www.efsa.europa.eu/en/pesticides/pesticidesscdocs.htm
European Chemical Substances Information System	http://ihcp.jrc.ec.europa.eu/our_databases/esis

Examples of this kind of authoritative evaluation are given in Table 1. Many can be accessed on the Internet, for example via the eChemPortal (http://www.echemportal.org) of the Organisation for Economic Co-operation and Development (OECD).

When an assessment based on an existing evaluation (probably for a different type of use) is being undertaken, any of the original study reports identified as critical to the risk assessment should also be consulted (where available): they may contain additional data relevant to the risk assessment for aircraft disinsection insecticides. Searches of the published literature and for unpublished data ("grey literature") should be carried out, in particular to identify any new data available; any relevant information identified should be evaluated and considered, as appropriate.

4.1.2 Types of health hazard data

Human data

In the case of insecticides that have been in use for many years, human data may be available. These data could include:

- results of epidemiological studies, including occupational studies on those manufacturing or using the pesticide formulations in question, or general population studies;
- ethically approved volunteer studies examining mild, temporary effects of short-term exposure or toxicokinetics of the substance in a limited number of subjects;
- case-reports of accidental and deliberate exposures and poisonings;
- health surveillance reports of exposed individuals;
- biomonitoring studies;
- clinical trials for human medicines, where an insecticide is being used or being considered for therapeutic use in humans;
- pharmacovigilance studies and adverse reaction monitoring when the chemical is used as a human medicine.

Evaluation of the relevance of these studies to risk assessment and their advantages and limitations are discussed in greater detail elsewhere (e.g. WHO, 1999; WHO, 2009). In general, however, existing reliable human data on toxicity should take precedence over animal data in the risk assessment. Hazard information data are most often available only for active ingredients, but all available data on the formulation should be noted.

Experimental toxicity data

For many pesticides, the human database is very limited and hazard assessment is dependent on information from experimental animals and in-vitro studies. For insecticides recently registered or reregistered for use by regulatory authorities, it is expected that comprehensive toxicology studies will have been conducted according to modern standards and good laboratory practice (GLP), using internationally accepted protocols for toxicity testing such as those published by OECD (OECD, 1987) or USEPA (http://www.epa.gov/ocspp/pubs/frs/home/guidelin.htm). For older pesticides, animal toxicity data may be limited and may not encompass modern requirements (unless they have been recently evaluated in regulatory programmes intended to review old pesticides).

Like other chemicals, insecticide formulations used in aircraft disinsection have the potential to cause a wide range of toxic effects. To identify the critical effects of the insecticide in question, a range of toxicity studies are usually needed. Although test requirements may vary to some extent with the country or region or with the precise use of the pesticide, the range of tests normally needed for health risk assessment, e.g. in regulatory approval of pesticides and biocides in OECD countries, is very similar (see Table 2).

It should be noted that toxicity test data are usually available only for pure substances – that is, for the active ingredients or solvents used in insecticide formulations rather than for the pesticide formulations themselves. In some jurisdictions, however, certain acute toxicity tests may also be performed with an insecticide formulation to establish labelling requirements and to ensure that the acute toxicity does not differ from that predicted on the basis of the tests on its individual components.

In the assessment of health risks of aircraft disinsection, local effects including irritation and sensitization will not be covered by the health-based guidance values, which are established on the basis of systemic effects. In aircraft disinsection, the skin-sensitizing properties of the chemicals will be important and can be assessed in animals in tests such as the guinea-pig maximization test, the Buehler test and, preferably, the local lymph node assay. Data on these tests should be available. No validated tests are available for testing respiratory tract sensitization; usually, however, respiratory tract sensitizers are positive in the above-mentioned skin sensitization tests. In addition, available human data on skin and respiratory tract sensitization should be checked and analysed.

Information on dermal absorption will be useful in the risk assessment of aircraft disinsection. Residual sprays are especially intended

Table 2. Range of toxicity tests normally required for pesticide approval

Toxicokinetic studies, usually in the rat, using single and repeat oral dosing, to give information on absorption, distribution, metabolism and excretion of the parent compound and its metabolites.
Acute toxicity studies to define the approximate lethal doses by oral, percutaneous, and sometimes inhalation routes, and the effects on body weight, clinical signs and gross pathology produced at lower dose levels following single-dose administration.
Skin and eye irritation studies
Skin sensitization studies
Repeat-dose oral toxicity studies*, normally for a minimum of 90 days in both rat and dog, to identify effects on organs, tissues, blood cells, and blood and urine chemical analytes.
Repeat-dose dermal and inhalation studies* of 28 or 90 days' duration may sometimes be required.
Genetic toxicity studies in vitro for gene mutation and chromosomal damage. If any in-vitro tests are indicative of positive results, in-vivo genetic toxicity studies should also be carried out.
Chronic oral toxicity and carcinogenicity studies*, in the rat and mouse, to assess long-term toxicity and effects on tumour incidence.
Reproductive toxicity studies*, including a multigeneration study in the rat and developmental toxicity studies in the rat and rabbit, to assess effects on male and female reproductive capacity and effects on embryonic/fetal development.
Delayed neurotoxicity studies are required for insecticides with structures related to those known to cause delayed neurotoxicity, such as organophosphates.
For more recently approved substances, studies of **acute and repeat-dose neurotoxicity***, **developmental neurotoxicity***, **dermal penetration** and **immunotoxicology*** and other specialized studies may have been performed.

Note: Studies marked with an asterisk (*) may provide useful dose–response information.

to deposit on the surfaces, and even though space treatment is not expected to leave any residual deposit, small droplets may be deposited on some surfaces within the aircraft to which passengers will be subsequently exposed. Further, inhalation toxicity studies may be of value in assessing risks to passengers, cabin crew members and ground operators, who are subject to potential acute and/or repeated inhalation exposure.

Absorption of the insecticide by inhalation, ingestion and through the skin should be estimated in the hazard assessment. If no chemical-specific data exist, which is often the case, default values should be used. For inhalation, a default value of 100% is assumed. For ingestion of insecticide during the exposure assessment, 100% will often be assumed as the default value, but the extent of bioavailability also needs to be taken into account when setting a tolerable systemic dose value from oral studies (see section 4.1.6). For dermal absorption of pyrethroids and of insecticides of other chemical structure with molecular mass >500 and octanol/water partition coefficient (log P_{ow})<−1 or >4, 10% is used as the default; for other insecticides, 100% is used (EC, 2002). It should be noted that ground service staff preparing spray solutions from a concentrated formulation may be exposed to both the undiluted formulation and to the product as sprayed, that is, as a diluted solution; others exposed to the spray are exposed only to the diluted solution. Dermal absorption may be different for these two. Thus, for preparation (mixing and loading) of spray solutions, the absorption rate of the undiluted formulation should be used; for other dermal exposure, the absorption rate of the diluted spray is more appropriate (EC, 2002; WHO, 2012b).

4.1.3 Evaluation of the toxicity information

An experienced toxicologist should evaluate the range and quality of human and animal toxicity information available. Although all the toxicity tests described in the previous section are useful for assessment of the hazard potential of an insecticide used for disinsection, it is recognized that not all such tests may have been performed, that not all the studies performed were of good quality, and that such data will therefore be valid for use in risk assessment only with restrictions. However, although good-quality studies may be missing for some toxic end-points, potential health hazards can often be characterized by weight-of-evidence analysis. It is especially important to recognize possible critical data gaps that may make the assessment uncertain. If the database is poor, information on chemically related compounds may be useful in the assessment.

The following points are of particular importance in evaluating the relevance of toxicological studies to hazard identification and risk assessment:

- Experimental design and quality of the critical study or studies. This includes, for example, purity of the active ingredient tested, physicochemical properties (stability, etc.), size of the study (number of exposure groups, group sizes, sex, etc.), suitability of the exposure levels used, duration of exposure, extent of toxicological and statistical evaluation, relevance of the route of exposure to humans, and whether the study adhered to established guidelines and GLP (WHO, 1999; WHO, 2009).

- Nature of the effects seen and their severity, and whether they would be reversible on cessation of exposure.
- The possibility of identifying a dose–response relationship, no-observed-adverse-effect-level (NOAEL) or other point of departure, and lowest-observed-adverse-effect-level (LOAEL).

4.1.4 Insecticides not recommended for use in aircraft disinsection

Compounds meeting the criteria of carcinogenicity, mutagenicity or reproductive toxicity categories 1A and 1B of the *Globally harmonized system of classification and labelling of chemicals* (UNECE, 2011) can be regarded as highly hazardous pesticides (JMPM, 2008). The Joint Meeting on Pesticide Management (JMPM) has issued a general recommendation that pesticides meeting the criteria for highly hazardous pesticides should not be registered for use unless:

– a clear need is demonstrated;
– there are no relevant alternatives based on risk–benefit analysis; and
– control measures, as well as good marketing practices, are sufficient to ensure that the product can be handled with acceptable risk to human health and the environment (JMPM, 2008).

It is suggested that this recommendation be followed in the case of aircraft disinsection as well. It is generally considered that compounds that are both genotoxic and carcinogenic are particularly likely to exert effects at very low doses: even if studies indicate apparent NOAELs, these products should not be used for aircraft disinsection.

It is also recommended that insecticides that produce clear reproductive toxic effects at dose levels causing no general toxicity are not used for aircraft disinsection. Among the exposed groups, unborn children, infants and toddlers – as well as older children – are of special concern because of their pattern of exposure and possible greater sensitivity to some toxic chemical actions. Fetal exposure is less of an issue for passengers than for aircrew since passengers are exposed on only a single occasion. Nevertheless, the possibility that an insecticide may induce developmental effects as a result of a single exposure must be considered.

Space spraying in aircraft disinsection involves exposure of the general public in circumstances in which respiratory protection cannot be effected and short-time exposure may be high. In general, therefore, products that can cause respiratory sensitization or reactions in previously sensitized individuals (identified from human cases or epidemiological studies) should not be used for this purpose. Since there are no validated animal tests for respiratory sensitization testing, the use of compounds that are positive in skin sensitization tests should also be considered carefully.

An insecticide of high acute toxicity, meeting the criteria of class Ia or Ib of the WHO Recommended Classification of Pesticides by Hazard (WHO, 2010), is not recommended for use in aircraft disinsection. However, it is the acute toxicity of the *formulation*, not just of the active ingredient, that should be taken into account, based on data relating to the formulation itself. If both the active insecticide ingredient and the formulation have been shown to cause a high incidence of severe or irreversible adverse effects on human health, use of that particular insecticide may not be acceptable (JMPM, 2008).

4.1.5 Other special considerations in hazard assessment

Interactions between insecticides and other constituents of the formulation

If two or more insecticides are used concurrently, possible toxicological interactions between those insecticides should be considered. Insecticides of the same class may produce dose-additive toxic effects; organophosphates, for example, reduce acetylcholinesterase activity. Other forms of interaction include synergistic (supra-additive) and antagonistic effects, which may be caused by different classes of pesticides, for example because of metabolic interactions. Unfortunately, reliable information is often unavailable, but knowledge of metabolic pathways or of receptor binding may sometimes help in identifying possible interactions.

Interactions may also occur between the active ingredient and the co-formulants used in the technical product. Moreover, impurities present in the technical product, e.g. in organophosphate products, may affect its final toxicity. Comprehensive specification of technical material (see http://www.who.int/whopes/quality/en/) is thus of the utmost importance. Available evidence of synergy at low doses is very limited (Meek et al., 2011).

The products used for aircraft disinsection may cause symptoms as a result of the odours or irritation caused by propellants and the solvents they contain. The risk assessment model does not cover these possible effects.

It is recognized that products registered for use in aircraft disinsection may also be subject to requirements relating to physical hazards (e.g. flammability, or corrosion of aircraft materials) that may restrict the solvents/propellants used. These requirements are outside the scope of this document.

It must also be noted that all insecticides used should be compliant with WHO specifications for public health pesticides (see http://www.who.int/whopes/quality/en/).

4.1.6 Dose–response assessment and setting of acceptable exposure levels

Dose–response assessment, with identification of a point of departure, is an essential part of hazard assessment for establishing health-based guidance values and for the assessment of risks. Different methods are available (WHO, 2009). The standard NOAEL approach can be regarded as a simplified form of dose–response analysis, identifying a single dose assumed to be without appreciable adverse effects (WHO, 2009). An important alternative approach is the benchmark dose method, based on the calculation of a benchmark dose at which a particular level of response would occur (WHO, 2009).

NOAEL approach

For the types of toxic effect caused by compounds considered acceptable for use for aircraft disinsection it is generally recognized that there is a dose or concentration below which adverse effects do not occur; for these, an NOAEL and/or LOAEL can be identified.

The NOAEL and LOAEL values are study-specific dose levels observed in animal or human studies. The NOAEL is the highest dose in a study at which no statistically significant adverse effect, compared with controls (or unexposed individuals), is observed, while the LOAEL is the lowest dose at which a statistically significant adverse effect is observed. The study design and the sensitivity of the test system can have a significant influence on NOAELs and LOAELs, which therefore represent only surrogates for the real no-effect and lowest-effect levels. Potentially relevant dose–response data and NOAELs/LOAELs for the purpose of establishing acceptable exposure levels can be obtained from repeated-dose toxicity studies, chronic toxicity/carcinogenicity studies, reproductive toxicity studies and some specialized toxicity studies. Human epidemiological studies, e.g. on occupationally exposed workers, may also provide useful dose–response data.

Different NOAELs/LOAELs are usually identified for different toxicities/end-points; they can be tabulated for each type of toxicity to help in identification of the critical end-point and the critical study. The lowest relevant NOAEL/LOAEL value should normally be used for risk characterization and the establishment of health-based guidance values. It should be noted, however, that the critical effects may not always be the same for different exposure scenarios. For example, for scenarios involving acute exposure to an acutely toxic insecticide, such as spraying of the insecticide, acute systemic effects and irritation may be the critical effects, whereas effects from repeated-dose/long-term/chronic studies should be considered in establishing acceptable exposure levels for long-term, low-level residual exposure. Exposure from residual sources will be predominantly via skin and hand–mouth contact, whereas acute exposure from spraying may be predominantly via inhalation. It should also be noted that, for many types of insecticide (e.g. carbamates, pyrethroids), the lowest NOAEL may be based on acute effects on the nervous system (independent of the overall length of the toxicity study).

The following additional points should be noted when identifying NOAELs/LOAELs for insecticides (WHO, 2010):

- If irreversible toxicity is noted in any organs at higher dose levels than that at which the critical effect occurs, these levels should also be noted in case they may be relevant to determining acceptable exposure levels or to prediction of possible additional risks that may be present if certain exposure levels are exceeded.
- The NOAEL is the highest dose tested without any statistically significant effect. However, there may be studies in which the lowest dose tested is a clear effect level and in which it is not possible to identify a NOAEL. In these cases, this lowest dose should be tabulated, noting that the LOAEL is the lowest dose tested. Alternatively, the method for the derivation of a benchmark dose could be used (see below).

Benchmark dose

When appropriate dose–response data are available, a benchmark dose (BMD) approach can be used as an alternative to the NOAEL for determining a point of departure for establishing health-based guidance values (WHO, 2009). In contrast to the NOAEL, which represents a single dose assumed to be without appreciable effect, the BMD is based on data from the entire dose–response curve of the critical effect (WHO, 2009). To take account of uncertainty in the experimental data, it is normal practice to use the lower 95% confidence limit on the BMD, i.e. the BMDL, as a point of departure.

Setting tolerable systemic doses: the use of uncertainty factors

The health-based guidance value (acceptable exposure level) used in this document is termed the tolerable systemic dose (TSD). In establishing TSD levels, critical NOAELs/LOAELs (or BMDLs) are divided by uncertainty factors (UFs) to account for variability and different uncertainties:

$$\text{TSD} = \text{N(L)OAEL/UF} \times F$$

where F represents the systemic bioavailability.

A TSD is usually expressed in mg absorbed chemical/kg body weight per day.

Uncertainty factors are necessary to take account of uncertainties in the database, of interspecies differences and of variability in the human population (interindividual differences). Unless there are chemical-specific data to support the use of chemical-specific UFs (WHO, 2005c), the use of default UFs to account for these uncertainties is a standard approach in the setting of TSDs. If the critical NOAEL (or BMDL) is derived from an animal study, a default UF of 10 is usually recommended to account for interspecies differences (WHO, 1994; WHO, 1999). A default UF of 10 is also used to account for interindividual differences in the general population (WHO, 1994; WHO, 1999). Contributors to the overall UF are normally multiplied because they are considered to be independent factors; the most commonly used default UF for the setting of TSDs for the general population is therefore 10 × 10 = 100 (WHO, 1994; WHO, 1999). However, this default approach can be modified if appropriate chemical-specific toxicokinetic or toxicodynamic data exist to justify different UFs for interspecies or interindividual differences. Further information on chemical-specific adjustment factors may be found elsewhere (WHO, 2005c).

In some cases, the use of additional UFs is justified (Dourson, Knauf & Swartout, 1992; Herrman & Younes, 1999; Vermeire, 1999; WHO, 1999; Dorne & Renwick, 2005; WHO, 2005c). Situations in which additional UFs should be considered include the following:

- When a LOAEL is used instead of an NOAEL, an additional UF (e.g. 3 or 10) is usually incorporated. This additional UF is based on expert judgement and will vary with the slope of the dose–response curve and the magnitude of the effect at the LOAEL.
- When an NOAEL from a sub-chronic study (in the absence of a chronic study) is used to derive a TSD for long-term exposure, an additional UF (commonly 2–10) is usually incorporated to take account of the attendant uncertainties.
- If the critical NOAEL relates to serious, irreversible toxicity, such as developmental abnormalities or cancer induced by a non-genotoxic mechanism, especially if the dose–response curve is steep (WHO, 1999). It is unlikely that an insecticide causing these effects would be acceptable for aircraft disinsection.
- When there are exposed subgroups that may be particularly sensitive to the effects of the compound (e.g. neonates because of

incompletely developed metabolism), and the available database does not adequately cover those subgroups.

- If the database is otherwise limited.
- If the NOAEL/LOAEL is derived from human data, the UF for interspecies differences is not necessary.

Types of tolerable systemic dose levels needed for the risk assessment of aircraft disinsection

Different reference values/TSDs may be needed according to the type of insecticide, its use pattern and the population of concern. In situations where there is repeated exposure, such as of those applying pesticides, the most relevant value is the TSD for long-term exposure, based on, for example, the acceptable daily intake (ADI). For insecticides with marked acute toxicity, however, it is important also to verify that the maximal daily exposure is acceptable; for this purpose the TSD for acute exposure, TSD_{AC} (based on, for example, the ARfD – acute reference dose) is used (Solecki et al., 2005).

Repeated exposure

For exposure of the passengers or cabin crew, a TSD for repeated insecticide exposure will be needed.

The long-term TSD is usually based on systemic effects observed in long-term studies and is expressed as mg/kg body weight per day. For most insecticides, values for long-term TSDs have already been established by international or national bodies based on, for example, ADIs set by JMPR/JECFA or by the European Union, reference doses or concentrations (RfDs, RfCs) set by USEPA, and minimal risk levels set by the ATSDR. While preference in the risk assessment for aircraft disinsection procedures should be the ADIs established by WHO, guidance values established by other authoritative bodies can be used, especially in the absence of WHO guidance values or when WHO guidance values no longer represent current knowledge.

Long-term TSDs are derived from oral studies: chronic studies most commonly use the oral route and many health-based guidance values, such as the ADIs set by JMPR, are intended primarily to control pesticide residue intake through the diet. In aircraft disinsection, however, operators and passengers are exposed predominantly via skin contact and inhalation. All exposure routes must therefore be taken into account in estimating the total systemic exposure. For a route-to-route extrapolation, the NOAEL from oral studies or the ADIs from JMPR/JECFA need to be corrected for oral bioavailability; this accounts for incomplete absorption and the possibility of first-pass effect (EC, 2006). Parent compounds absorbed into the circulation of the gut are rapidly transported to the liver and may be extensively metabolized before reaching the systemic circulation (and possible target organs). Thus, systemic concentrations of parent compounds may be higher following dermal or inhalation exposure than following oral exposure.

Information about oral bioavailability is not always directly available. Based on the entire toxicity database, including information on physicochemical properties, a value for oral bioavailability needs to be derived; for example, when the median lethal dose (LD_{50}) values for a dermal and an oral acute study are of the same order, it is likely that dermal and oral absorption are also of the same order. If a default value is to be used in the absence of any information allowing a specific value to be derived, it should be noted that selecting a value of 100% oral bioavailability does not represent a conservative approach: the default value selected should reflect the degree of caution required.

During application of insecticides, both the individuals spraying and the aircraft passengers may be at risk of inhalation exposure. It is therefore critical to ensure that the insecticide has no significant local respiratory effects and that TSDs for long-term systemic exposure are also protective against possible respiratory effects.

Regional and national occupational exposure levels (OELs) may be available for public health pesticides. However, it should be noted that these values do not take into account skin exposure, which may be more significant than inhalation exposure in pesticide application. In addition, OELs are usually set on the assumption that the insecticide is used by adult, healthy workers, exposed only for the duration of the working day or for shorter periods of time, and may thus reflect only the need to protect against local effects such as irritation. The UFs applied in setting OELs therefore tend to be much smaller than those used in setting guidelines for population exposure. For personnel applying insecticides, TSDs should not be based on national or regional OELs. Some jurisdictions have established "Acceptable Operator Exposure Levels" (AOELs) for pesticides, which take account of all routes of exposure and are expressed as a systemic dose. These AOEL values could therefore be used as a starting point for establishing TSDs for insecticides used in aircraft disinsection.

It is recommended that the same TSDs be used for operators and for passengers.

Short-term exposure

Health-based guidance values for short-term (24-hour) exposure have been established by JMPR for insecticides with presumed significant acute toxicity, such as acutely neurotoxic insecticides, including those with anticholinesterase activity (organophosphates and carbamates); these values are called "Acute Reference Doses" (ARfD).

The ARfD is defined as the amount of a chemical, expressed on a body weight basis, that can be ingested over a short period of time, such as one day, without appreciable risk to health (JMPR, 1998; Solecki et al., 2005). It is established similarly to the long-term ADI, using relevant human or animal studies of acute or short-term dosing. The critical NOAEL from such studies is used to establish the ARfD by application of a UF. If the data derive from animal studies, an overall UF of 100 is quite commonly used unless chemical-specific information is available to support the use of a lower UF as described above (Solecki et al., 2010).

4.2 Exposure assessment

4.2.1 *Measured data from the scientific literature*

The WHO publication *Safety of pyrethroids for public health use* (WHO, 2005b) summarizes several studies that provide data on exposure to pyrethroids from various public health scenarios, including aircraft disinsection (Sutton, 2003; Berger-Preiss et al., 2004). Further exposure studies are available that include sampling of residues on surfaces, concentrations in air and dermal exposure of the spray operator following spraying within aircraft (Berger-Preiss et al., 2006; Sutton et al., 2007). A biomonitoring study by Wei et al. (2011) involved measuring metabolites of pyrethroids in the urine of a self-selected group of flight attendants.

None of the available exposure studies permits a correlation to be made directly between body burden and the amount of pesticide sprayed. Numbers of samples were generally small, in some cases there are uncertainties regarding timing of sampling relative to exposure, and some sampling was performed only on a "spot sample" basis.

4.2.2 Modelling approach

The ability of a pesticide to cause adverse health effects depends on the toxicity of the insecticide, the route of exposure (ingestion, inhalation, dermal contact), the frequency and duration of exposure and the inherent sensitivity of the exposed person. Exposure assessment of aircraft disinsection procedures therefore consists of several different scenarios for different target groups. Exposure has been assumed to be strongly related to the actual amount of product or active ingredient handled and applied.

For the risk characterization, a total exposure estimate must be calculated by summing up all relevant exposure routes and pathways.

The exposure assessment described in this document should be considered as a first-tier approach. Whenever needed, higher-tier assessments with more complex methods should be used. For example, probabilistic risk assessment with quantification of uncertainties can be used to estimate risks in more detail. WHO has published guidance on exposure models and communicating uncertainties (WHO, 2008). The defaults should be modified by the user of the models on a case-by-case basis and replaced with appropriate measured or otherwise improved point values or distributions, when applicable.

It is the aim of this document to provide an estimate of the risks in:

- optimal conditions, i.e. the guideline scenario; and
- a lax standard scenario, which allows for some common deviations from the instructions and, in some cases, for exposures that are accidental by nature.

Incidents such as severe malfunctioning of equipment (significant leaks, problems with spray pressure, equipment whose outer surface is heavily contaminated with the insecticide) may lead to very high exposure by both inhalation and dermal routes. For instance a larger area of skin than normal may be exposed, or inhalation exposure may be greater because incorrect spray pressure changes the characteristics of the spray. These situations are not covered in this risk assessment.

The models follow the WHO guidance provided in *A generic risk assessment model for insecticide-treated nets* (WHO, 2012b) and other current public health pesticide model development work by WHO. For assessing inhalation exposure to aerosols sprayed from cans (i.e. space spraying), the ConsExpo model (Delmaar, Park & van Engelen, 2005; Delmaar & Bremmer, 2009), developed by the National Institute for Public Health and the Environment (RIVM) in the Netherlands, is used. This mathematical model represents a way of modelling both consumer exposure and, in suitable cases, worker exposure. Particularly when aircraft cabin crew handle insecticides in aerosol spray cans, use of consumer models is justified (rather than considering cabin crew as professional operators). The ConsExpo model is well established, widely used and accepted among regulatory authorities for assessing biocidal products. The model is also recommended by the European Chemicals Agency for REACH registration purposes in first- and higher-tier risk assessments.

4.2.3 General parameters for exposure assessment

Procedures for indoor application of residual insecticides, including residual disinsection, are presented in detail in a WHO manual (WHO, 2007); WHO has also published specifications for compression sprayers used in such applications (WHO, 2006). A practitioner's guide for space spraying published by WHO describes in detail the appropriate spraying equipment and other issues that must be considered for safe and effective application of space spray products (WHO, 2003). More aircraft-specific guidance and information about the practices have also been published by WHO (1995; 2005b) and, on a national level, by the governments of Australia and New Zealand in the Schedule of Aircraft Disinsection Procedures (DAFF/MPI, 2012).

Anthropometric parameters

Anthropometric and physiological parameters (e.g. body weight, skin surface area, respiration rates) all have an effect on risk estimates. If data are derived from a published database, it is preferable that the database be internally consistent: all needed parameters for all age groups should be available and derived from the same population. Databases produced in the USA (USEPA, 2008; USEPA, 2011) are extensive and up to date, cover all age groups and all relevant anthropometric and physiological data, and have been used as the source of data used in this document.

Ground personnel, cabin crew members and adult passengers are assumed to weigh 62 kg (adult female mean – taken as protective of both sexes, USEPA, 2011) (Table 3).

Risks are also estimated for children aged 11–16 years (assumed to weigh 32 kg), toddlers, i.e. children aged 2–3 years (14 kg), and newborns (4.8 kg) (50th percentile, birth to 1 month; USEPA, 2008).

The film thickness of a non-viscous liquid likely to be in contact with unprotected, immersed skin is assumed to be 0.01 cm after run-off. For use of an aerosol spray it is estimated that the area of fingers exposed will be one-tenth of the surface area of the hands (total surface area of hands = 930 cm^2; USEPA, 2011). Thus, the maximum amount of liquid on exposed fingers will be 1 ml.

The area of skin potentially exposed to insecticide reflects the clothing worn. It is assumed that the skin areas exposed to insecticide residues after residual spraying is 50% of the hands and forearms for cabin crew and 50% of the hands, forearms, lower legs and feet for passengers (sitting position, adults and older children). The body surface areas for different age groups are presented in Table 3. The total exposed area is 0.1 m^2 for the cabin crew, 0.25 m^2 for adult passengers and 0.16 m^2 for children aged 6–11 years. Younger children

Table 3. Anthropometric and physiological characteristics used in the model[a]

	Adult[b]	Child 6–11 years	Toddler 2–3 years	Newborn[c]
Weight (kg)	62	32	14	4.8
Body surface (m^2)				
total	1.69	1.05	0.61	0.29
hands	0.093	0.054	0.032	0.015
arms	0.265	0.137	0.072	0.040
forearms	0.088[d]	0.059[e]	0.035[f]	0.017[f]
legs	0.556	0.301	0.142	0.060
lower legs	0.199[g]	0.125[h]	0.066[i]	0.031[i]
feet	0.123	0.078	0.043	0.019
head	0.135	0.136	0.087	0.053
trunk	0.556	0.375	0.235	0.104
Respiration rate (m^3/h)[j]				
sleep/nap	0.40	0.38	0.38	0.28[k]
sedentary	0.40	0.38	0.40	0.28[k]
light activity	0.89	0.90	1.0	0.66[k]
moderate activity	1.9	1.7	1.7	1.3[k]

[a] Source: USEPA, 2008; USEPA, 2011
[b] 16–21 years, female
[c] Birth to 1 month
[d] 5.2% of the whole body surface (USEPA, 2011)
[e] 5.5% of the whole body surface (USEPA, 2011)
[f] 5.7% of the whole body surface (USEPA, 2011)
[g] 11.7% of the whole body surface (USEPA, 2011)
[h] 12.5% of the whole body surface (USEPA, 2011)
[i] 11.7% of the whole body surface (USEPA, 2011)
[j] 95th percentile of the activity category
[k] Birth to 1 year

(toddlers), aged 2–3 years, may be more active and, as a worst-case assumption, one-third of the whole skin area of 0.61 m^2 may be exposed, i.e. an exposure area of 0.2 m^2. For direct exposures to space spraying applications of insecticide, the surface areas assumed to be exposed are the head and 50% of the hands, forearms and lower legs. Thus, the total exposed area is 0.33 m^2 for adults, 0.26 m^2 for children aged 6–11 years and 0.15 m^2 for toddlers.

It is estimated that 11% of the insecticide on contact surfaces is transferred onto skin (95th percentile for hard surfaces – USEPA, 2009).

Toddlers are prone to mouthing different objects and may well ingest dust from contaminated hands. It is estimated that 10% of material on skin goes from hands to mouth (USEPA, 2009). The hand area of a child aged 2–3 years is 0.032 m^2 (USEPA, 2008).

It is assumed that the skin of newborn infants is not exposed to insecticide on aircraft surfaces, as they are held, transported in their own carriers or are otherwise covered with clothing, with very limited opportunity for contact with aircraft surfaces.

Default values for respiration rates are: 0.4 m^3/hour for resting adults (passengers), 0.89 m^3/hour for adults performing light activities (cabin crew), 1.9 m^3/hour for adults performing moderate activities (spray operators), 0.38 m^3/hour for children and toddlers at rest and 0.28 m^3/hour for newborn infants (USEPA, 2011).

Parameters for assessment of ground operator exposure – residual disinsection

Recommended sprayed amounts, active ingredient concentrations of products, and other product- and chemical-specific information should be obtained from product labels, material safety data sheets and product instruction manuals.

It is assumed that residual spraying is carried out by trained ground personnel, not by cabin crew. In this exposure assessment, the guideline scenario assumes compliance with both WHO recommendations and product label instructions. Product label instructions can include the use of personal protective equipment (PPE) to protect against exposure, for example protective clothing or gloves. Respiratory protective equipment is often recommended when spraying is done in enclosed spaces. For indoor residual spraying, which is a similar scenario, WHO recommends that coveralls are worn. In the lax standard scenario, it is assumed that no actual personal protection equipment is used– only normal light clothing covering the trunk, etc. but, for example, no gloves. The spray equipment in that scenario may not be fully leakproof, its outer surface may have been contaminated earlier, the spray pressure may be intermittently high, etc., as defined below in the specific exposure scenarios. The tasks that are considered to cause exposure to the workers are:

- mixing and loading;
- application of the insecticide product by spraying; and
- washing and maintenance of the spray equipment.

Parameters for assessment of cabin crew exposure – space spraying

It is assumed that space spraying is performed by the aircraft crew using disposable pressurized cans of the insecticide and that there is therefore no mixing or loading. No actual personal protection is assumed; only normal light clothing covering the trunk, etc. but, for example, no gloves. Thus the guideline scenario is similar to the lax standard scenario.

4.2.4 Algorithms used to estimate exposure and absorbed dose from residual spraying of aircraft disinsection products

It should be emphasized that chemical-specific or case-specific data should always be sought and used when possible.

Ground personnel (operator) exposure

This scenario considers adults exposed only via direct dermal and inhalation routes. Formulations used for residual spraying are prepared by mixing the product with water to reach a product-specific concentration specified in the use instructions. Quantities depend on the area of interior surfaces of the aircraft cabin and cargo compartments. The required dosage per square metre is also chemical-specific. After spraying, any material should be cleared from the air by running the air-conditioning for at least for one hour.

Mixing and loading insecticide formulation

In mixing and loading, only dermal exposure is considered significant. It is assumed that the amount of the spray liquid prepared per day is three 10-litre tanks (sufficient to treat a large aircraft). It is also assumed that ground personnel treating aircraft need to spray aeroplanes twice a week throughout the year. Default values for potential hand contamination (ml/operation) during mixing and

Table 4. Default values for potential hand contamination (ml/operation) during mixing and loading of a liquid pesticide formulation (no gloves used[a])

Size of container and diameter of opening	Contamination of hands (ml/operation)
1 litre, any closure	0.01
2 litres, any closure	0.01
5 litres, narrow closure	0.2
5 litres, 45 mm or 63 mm closure	0.01
10 litres, narrow closure	0.5
10 litres, 45 mm closure	0.1
10 litres, 63 mm closure	0.05
20 litres, narrow closure	0.5
20 litres, 63 mm closure	0.05

[a] Contamination arising from solid formulations is described in WHO, 2011a.

Source: CRD, 2007.

loading of a liquid pesticide formulation (without the use of gloves) are adapted from the UK POEM model and are shown in Table 4 (CRD, 2007). For small packages (1–2 litres), the contamination is estimated to be 0.01 ml/operation. In the lax standard scenario, it is assumed that no gloves are worn. In the guideline scenario (i.e. working according to WHO and label recommendations), the use of gloves is assumed, giving 90% protection.

$$\text{Predicted dose} = \frac{VF_{\text{dermal}} \times CF \times PPE \times AbsD \times EF}{BW \times AT}$$

where:

Predicted dose = systemic dose due to dermal exposure from liquid formulations, mg a.i./kg body weight per day (TWA – time-weighted average)

VF_{dermal} = volume of formulation on hands (0.01 ml/operation, from CRD (2007)) × no. of daily operations (3)

CF = concentration of active ingredient in the formulation (chemical-specific data), mg/ml

PPE = factor to reflect reduction of exposure due to use of gloves (0.1 for guideline scenario, 1.0 for lax standard scenario)

$AbsD$ = dermal absorption of the non-diluted formulation (default for pyrethroids, 10%; for others, see section 4.1.2)

EF = exposure frequency, 2 days/week, 52 weeks per year (104 days)

BW = body weight (62 kg)

AT = averaging time, 1 year (365 days)

Even though highly acutely toxic insecticides are not recommended for use for aircraft disinsection, acute neurotoxicity is the most sensitive end-point in the case of some insecticides. In these cases, therefore, the acute exposure must also be calculated and compared with a health-based guidance value for acute exposure. This is also true for compounds that are otherwise acutely toxic, on the basis that there is need for an ARfD. The following equation is given as an example of a calculation of predicted acute systemic dose.

$$\text{Predicted acute dose} = \frac{VF_{\text{dermal}} \times CF \times PPE \times AbsD}{BW}$$

Application of insecticide formulation, washing and maintenance of the spray equipment, inhalation exposure

Even though this scenario relates to the treatment of surfaces, it is also necessary to consider inhalation exposure because a proportion of the insecticide aerosol (small droplets) will persist in the air. It is assumed that 0.1% of the active ingredient sprayed will be evenly distributed in the air, including the breathing zone of the operator. This value is derived by expert judgement and the user of the model is encouraged to use more specific defaults when available.

$$\text{Predicted dose} = \frac{Conc \times AR \times 0.001 \times RPE \times BV \times AbsP \times EF}{VOL \times BW \times AT}$$

where:

Predicted dose = systemic dose due to inhalation exposure to the spray, mg a.i./kg body weight per day (TWA).

$Conc$ = target concentration of the a.i. on surfaces in mg/m^2, i.e. product-specific target concentration of a.i. per unit area

AR = surface area to be treated (default, 2500 m^2– large aircraft assumed)

0.001 = factor for proportion of a.i. evenly distributed in the air (0.1%)

RPE = factor for reduction of exposure due to respiratory protective equipment (0.1 for guideline scenario, 1.0 for lax standard scenario)

BV = breathing volume (total amount of air breathed during the exposure, mean value for adults during moderate activities 1.9 m^3/h; assuming 2 hours spent in actual spraying during a workday, total volume of contaminated air breathed per day is 3.8 m^3

AbsP = absorption from the respiratory tract (default, 100%)

EF = exposure frequency, 2 days/week, 52 weeks per year (104 days)

VOL = volume of the aircraft (default 1000 m^3 – large aircraft assumed)

BW = body weight (62 kg)

AT = averaging time, 1 year (365 days)

If necessary, the acute systemic dose can also be calculated using the same equation but omitting the terms for exposure frequency (*EF*) and averaging time (*AT*).

Application of insecticide formulation, washing and maintenance of the spray equipment, dermal exposure

In a lax standard scenario, hands are exposed to the spray aerosol during application, and to the spray liquid during washing and maintenance of the equipment. The assumption has been made for the application of spray by hand-held equipment that exposure will be primarily to the hands, with other areas of the body receiving relatively minor doses. This assumption is supported by data from another exposure assessment model (the Bayesian Exposure Assessment Model (BEAT) – HSL, 2011)[1].

[1] The BEAT "PHI liquids" scenario data (collated from Llewellyn et al., 1996) cover insecticide being applied as low-pressure sprays in an overhead and downwards direction, i.e. analogous to the disinsection scenario. Potential exposures of the hands significantly exceed exposures of other areas of the body.

In the guideline scenario, the sprayer is fully leakproof, clothing that protects against the insecticide aerosol, e.g. overall and hat, is worn, and appropriate gloves are used both during the spraying and for washing and maintenance of the equipment. The protection factor of appropriately used protective clothing is 90%.

$$\text{Predicted dose} = \frac{VS_{\text{dermal}} \times CS \times PPE \times AbsD \times EF}{BW \times AT}$$

where:

Predicted dose = systemic dose due to dermal exposure, mg a.i./kg body weight per day (TWA)

VS_{dermal} = volume of spray on hands = 9.3 ml during the day (see section 4.2.3)

CS = concentration of a.i. in the spray (mg/ml), derived from concentration of a.i. in the formulation and its dilution for spraying

PPE = factor for reduction of exposure due to use of protective clothing (0.1 for guideline scenario, 1.0 for lax standard scenario)

EF = exposure frequency, 2 days/week, 52 weeks per year (104 days)

$AbsD$ = dermal absorption of the spray (diluted formulation) (default for pyrethroids, 10%; for others, see section 4.1.2)

BW = body weight (62 kg)

AT = averaging time, 1 year (365 days)

If necessary, the acute systemic dose can also be calculated using the same equation but omitting the terms for exposure frequency (EF) and averaging time (AT).

Cabin crew exposure

The on-flight cabin crew may also be exposed to residual sprays via skin when touching treated surfaces. There are estimated to be typically 20 air crew flight days per month, which means a maximum exposure duration of 240 days per year. Half of the exposed skin area (hands and forearms) is exposed (see section 4.2.3).

Since the product sprayed on surfaces has to be continuously effective against the particular pests, it is assumed that the target concentration is always available on the surfaces, regardless of the time elapsed since the most recent spraying.

$$\text{Predicted dose} = \frac{Conc \times P \times ESA \times AbsD \times EF}{BW \times AT}$$

where:

Predicted dose = systemic dose due to dermal exposure, mg a.i./kg body weight per day (TWA)

Conc = target concentration of a.i. on surfaces (mg/m^2), i.e. product-specific target concentration of a.i. per unit area

P = proportion translodged onto skin = 11% of the amount present on the surfaces (USEPA, 2009)

ESA = exposed skin area (0.1 m^2, i.e. 50% of hands and forearms)

AbsD = dermal absorption of the spray (diluted formulation) (default for pyrethroids, 10%; for others, see section 4.1.2)

EF = exposure frequency (default 240 days/year)

BW = body weight (62 kg)

AT = averaging time, 1 year (365 days)

If necessary, the acute systemic dose can also be calculated using the same equation but omitting the terms for exposure frequency (EF) and averaging time (*AT*).

Passenger exposure

Passengers include adults, children, toddlers and newborn infants. Passengers are assumed not to be exposed by inhalation after residual spraying, as aircrafts are well ventilated after treatment. Passenger exposure is assumed to be due to dermal exposure from the surfaces of the aircraft. In addition, the sprayed insecticide may be dislodged from surfaces as contaminated dust, leading to ingestion by toddlers through hand-to-mouth behaviour. It is assumed that newborn infants are not in contact with treated surfaces.

Dermal exposure – touching of treated surfaces; potential residues on toddlers' hands leading to hand-to-mouth ingestion exposure

The primary targets of spraying include areas under the seats, lower seat backs, overhead lockers and floors. It is assumed that the body parts most likely to be exposed are hands, legs and possibly feet. Since seats are not usually sprayed directly, dermal exposure to the remainder of the body via the seats is expected to be negligible, although there would be some incidental contamination. For toddlers, because of their more active behaviour, it is assumed that one-third of the whole skin is exposed.

As a worst-case situation, it is assumed that cabin surfaces have been treated only recently and that there has been no decay or decomposition of the active ingredient.

$$\text{Predicted dose} = \frac{Conc \times P \times ESA \times AbsD \times EF}{BW \times AT}$$

where:

Predicted dose = systemic dose due to dermal exposure, mg a.i./kg body weight per day (TWA)

Conc = target concentration of a.i. on surfaces (mg/m^2, i.e. product-specific target concentration of a.i. per unit area

P = proportion translodged onto skin = 11% of the amount present on the surfaces (USEPA, 2009)

ESA = exposed skin area (0.25 m^2 for adults, 0.16 m^2 for older children, 0.2 m^2 for toddlers); for toddlers, additionally, some of the insecticide on the hands is transported to the mouth by hand-to-mouth activity, leading to ingestion exposure (see next section).

AbsD = dermal absorption of the spray (diluted formulation) (default for pyrethroids, 10%; for others, see section 4.1.2)

EF = exposure frequency (default for adults (business travel), 40 days/year; for all children (e.g. holiday travel), 5 days/year)

BW = body weight (adults 62 kg, older children 32 kg, toddlers 14 kg)

AT = averaging time, 1 year (365 days)

If necessary, the acute systemic dose can also be calculated using the same equation but omitting the terms for exposure frequency (EF) and averaging time (*AT*).

Ingestion exposure of toddlers due to hand-to-mouth activity

Insecticide is transferred to the hands from the surfaces contacted (see above); the relevant hand area for toddlers is 0.032 m^2. For the extent of hand-to-mouth transfer, a default of 10% can be used.

$$\text{Predicted dose} = \frac{Conc \times P \times ESA \times THM \times AbsO \times EF}{BW \times AT}$$

where:

Predicted dose = systemic dose due to hand-to mouth transfer, mg a.i./kg body weight per day (TWA)

Conc = target concentration of a.i. on surfaces (mg/m^2), i.e. product-specific target concentration of a.i. per unit area

P = proportion translodged onto skin = 11% of the amount present on the surfaces (USEPA, 2009)

ESA = exposed skin area (0.032 m^2)

THM = extent of transfer from hands to mouth (10%)

AbsO = gastrointestinal absorption (default, 100%)

EF = exposure frequency (default, 5 days/year)

BW = body weight (14 kg)

AT = averaging time, 1 year (365 days)

If necessary, the acute systemic dose can also be calculated using the same equation but omitting the terms for exposure frequency (EF) and averaging time (*AT*).

4.2.5 Algorithms used to estimate exposure and absorbed dose caused by space spraying of aircraft disinsection products

Cabin crew exposure during spraying

This section considers cabin crew exposed via dermal and inhalation routes while spraying with aerosol cans. The insecticide formulation is packed into an aerosol can containing a propellant approved for use in aircraft. The aerosol can must be able to deliver an even distribution of spray (the 1995 WHO Consultation referred to a discharge rate of 1 gram per second). Mass median droplet diameter should be 8 μm (range 3–10 μm). The WHO document (WHO, 1995) gives detailed instructions for the spraying procedure in different types (and sizes) of aircraft. The Boeing 747 is used as an example: it may require a total of four 100-g cans to be completely emptied during the procedure to achieve the chemical-specific target concentration per cubic metre. The spray is applied as near the ceiling as possible by two members of the crew, each holding two cans and moving at a slow walking pace (one step or one seat row per second).

Space spraying for aircraft disinsection can take place before flight, before the passengers board the aircraft and/or during the flight with passengers on board. Only cabin personnel will be exposed to spray during pre-flight procedures, but both passengers and cabin crew will be exposed during flight; the exposures may therefore need to be summed for cabin crew. However, these treatments may be performed with different active ingredients, which further complicates the assessment.

Spraying the aerosol

It has been estimated, as a default, that the frequency of spraying is once per work day, i.e. 240 events per year. It must be remembered, however, that spraying schemes can be very different in different countries, and that the length of the air routes worked has an impact on the frequency with which cabin crew carry out spraying. Default spray duration is 200 seconds, and the exposure duration is 30 minutes. As reported by Berger-Preiss et al. (2004), more than 90% of the total amount inhaled is inhaled within the first 5–10 minutes after spraying. It is assumed that no respiratory protective equipment is used.

Three features of spraying aerosol cans in aircraft disinsection are untypical of spraying of aerosol products and therefore have an impact on the development of models for inhalation exposure:

- The air inside an operating aircraft is subject both to recirculation systems and to temperature control (air-conditioning). The distribution and dispersal of aerosols may not be the same as that in still air in a normal room. The air-circulation systems can be operated at different settings, and different parts of the aircraft experience different levels of ventilation, which can vary with aircraft type. There is also no consistent practice regarding how the ventilation system is operated. Calculations of rates of dilution of aircraft air by partial exhaustion and partial recirculation would be complex, and would differ by aircraft type. For these reasons, as a conservative estimate, no effect of ventilation will be assumed.
- Aerosol sprays for aircraft disinsection are available as both "multi-shot" and "one-shot" sprays. The "one-shot" sprays discharge their entire contents as a single continuous spray once the nozzle has been activated. This results in a different spray duration from what is generally the case for aerosol products, for which it is assumed that the operator does not continuously activate the nozzle. Assumptions in standard models regarding spray duration and discharge rates may not apply and situation-specific data may be needed. Adjustment may also be needed for the situation on an aircraft in which two spray cans may be operated simultaneously by one crew member, which may not reflect the default assumptions in aerosol spray models.
- When determining the amount of product sprayed, it is possible that the actual quantity sprayed may differ from the recommended doses. In some aircraft, the cabin volume is not a simple multiple of the volume that can be treated with one spray can, and an extra part-can would need to be used. However, it is likely that the full volume of each can supplied will in fact be emptied on each occasion (and this is unavoidable with one-shot cans), and a degree of overdosing can therefore be expected in these situations; this should be taken into account in the exposure assessment.

The ConsExpo spray model (Delmaar, Park & van Engelen, 2005; Delmaar & Bremmer, 2009) is a software model available in English, free of charge, via the Internet (www.consexpo.nl). Results can be obtained both as point estimates (as in this first-tier assessment) or as distributions, and the model calculations are all published in the model manual. The model can therefore be considered as transparent. Development work is continuous; the example calculations presented in this report were made with version 4.1.

An estimation of particle-size distribution is also available, should it be needed. The algorithms are presented in detail in the manual (Delmaar, Park & van Engelen, 2005); in this document, only some parts of the calculations are shown.

Inhalation exposure

ConsExpo 4.1 (Delmaar, Park & van Engelen, 2005; Delmaar & Bremmer, 2009) models indoor air concentration over time for slowly evaporating or non-volatile compounds in droplets released from a spray can. Using the modelled air concentration with information on breathing rate, exposure time and other exposure factors allows inhalation exposure to be determined. The exposure frequencies are similar to other scenarios, e.g. 240 times per year for cabin personnel.

The general exposure parameters needed include the spray duration (in this case estimated as 200 seconds), exposure duration (30 minutes), room volume (or, in this case, cabin volume; large aircraft default, 1000 m^3), room height (estimated 2 m), and ventilation rate (in this case it is assumed that there is no effect due to ventilation). A large aircraft is estimated to have an internal surface area of approximately 2500 m^2, including internal fittings.

The product-specific parameters required by the model for calculating the air concentration and inhalation uptake are as follows:

– mass generation rate, or the amount of compound released from one can during spraying per unit of time (default, 1 gram/second); this value needs to be increased if multiple cans are discharged simultaneously;
– estimated airborne, non-volatile fraction (assumed to be 100% as a worst-case assumption);
– weight fraction of non-volatiles (default, 2%);

- weight fraction of the compound of interest in the product (percentage of active ingredient in the product), from the product label;
- density of non-volatile compounds (assumed, 1.8 g/cm^3);
- initial particle distribution, assumed to be log-normal, average particle diameter 8 μm, coefficient of variation 0.45 μm;
- inhalation cut-off droplet diameter (15 μm);
- non-respirable uptake fraction (10%);
- respirable uptake fraction, assumed to be known from experimental studies (default, 100%)
- concentration of compound of interest in the (inhaled) air (kg/m^3, calculated above);
- inhalation rate of the exposed person (default mean value for adults during light activities (USEPA, 2008), 0.89 m^3/h);
- exposure time (default, 30 minutes).

The algorithms used to calculate air concentration can be found in the ConsExpo manual (www.consexpo.nl).

The ConsExpo model provides as output (among other formats) the internal inhalation dose (systemic exposure arising from the inhalation route) for acute (one event) and chronic (daily average) scenarios, per kilogram body weight based on the body weight value entered for the population of interest.

Dermal exposure

In the guideline scenario, the spray can is fully leakproof, appropriate gloves are used during the spraying when required, and the spraying procedure is performed as described by WHO (WHO, 1995) and according to label instructions.

Space spraying is intended to knock down flying insects but the spray is likely to deposit on the aircraft surfaces to some extent. It is assumed, however, that the deposited concentration is quite low and represents 1% of the material sprayed into the air at the required spray rates; the remainder is assumed to be removed by ventilation rather than by deposition on surfaces, although the rate of removal is not calculated because of differing ventilation practices.

$$\text{Predicted dose} = \frac{C \times P \times ESA \times EF \times AbsD}{BW \times AT}$$

where:

Predicted dose = systemic dose due to dermal exposure to surfaces, mg a.i./kg body weight per day (TWA)

C = concentration on the surface (calculated as 1% of the amount of active ingredient sprayed (product-specific information) divided by the internal surface area of the aircraft)

P = proportion translodged onto skin = 11% of the amount present on the surfaces (USEPA, 2009).

ESA = exposed skin area (0.1 m^2, i.e. 50% of hands and forearms)

EF = exposure frequency (default, 240 days/year).

$AbsD$ = dermal absorption of the spray (diluted formulation) (default for pyrethroids, 10%; for others, see section 4.1.2)

BW = body weight (62 kg)

AT = averaging time, 1 year (365 days)

In the lax standard scenario, fingers are exposed to the spray aerosol as a result of leaking at the nozzle of the aerosol can; gloves are not used or they are not appropriate for the purpose. This exposure is additional to the exposure calculated from contact with surfaces.

$$\text{Predicted dose} = \frac{VS_{\text{dermal}} \times CS \times EF \times AbsD}{BW \times AT}$$

where:

Predicted dose = systemic dose due to dermal exposure to spray on hands, mg a.i./kg body weight per day (TWA)

VS_{dermal} = volume of spray on fingers = 1 ml during the day (one-tenth of the amount on hands, as described in section 4.2.3)

CS = concentration a.i. in the spray (mg/ml, chemical-specific data)

EF = exposure frequency (default 240 days/year)

$AbsD$ = dermal absorption of the spray (diluted formulation) (default for pyrethroids, 10%; for others, see section 4.1.2)

BW = body weight (62 kg)

AT = averaging time, 1 year (365 days)

Finger (spray) and hand and forearm (surface) exposures are summed when calculating total exposure in the lax standard scenario.

If necessary, the acute systemic dose can also be calculated using the same equations but omitting the terms for exposure frequency (EF) and averaging time (AT).

Passenger exposure

Passengers include adults, children, toddlers and infants.

Indirect dermal exposure (passengers not present during space spraying)

The deposited concentration on surfaces is assumed to represent 1% of the target amount in the air.

$$\text{Predicted dose} = \frac{C \times P \times ESA \times EF \times AbsD}{BW \times AT}$$

where:

Predicted dose = systemic dose due to dermal exposure, mg a.i./kg body weight per day (TWA)

C = concentration on the surface (calculated as 1% of the amount of a.i. sprayed (product-specific information) divided by the aircraft internal surface area)

P = proportion translodged onto skin = 11% of the amount present on surfaces

ESA = exposed skin areas (0.25 m^2 for adults, 0.16 m^2 for older children, 0.2 m^2 for toddlers)

EF = exposure frequency (default for adults (business travel), 40 days/year; for all children (e.g. holiday travel), 5 days/year)

AbsD = dermal absorption of the spray (diluted formulation) (default for pyrethroids, 10%; for others, see section 4.1.2)

BW = body weight (adults 62 kg, older children 32 kg, toddlers 14 kg)

AT = averaging time, 1 year (365 days)

Inhalation exposure (passengers present during space spraying)

The approach used in the section on cabin crew exposure assessment is also applied for passengers. Different breathing volumes (activity-related), exposure frequencies and body weights must be taken into account.

Direct dermal exposure (passengers present during space spraying)

$$\text{Predicted dose} = \frac{C \times ESA \times EF \times AbsD}{BW \times AT}$$

where:

Predicted dose = systemic dose due to dermal exposure, mg a.i./kg body weight per day (TWA)

C = concentration settling on surfaces, including exposed skin (calculated as 1% of the amount of a.i. sprayed (product-specific information) divided by the aircraft internal surface area)

ESA = exposed skin areas (0.33 m^2 for adults, 0.26 m^2 for older children, 0.15 m^2 for toddlers)

EF = exposure frequency (default for adults (business travel), 40 days/year; for all children (e.g. holiday travel), 5 days/year)

AbsD = dermal absorption of the spray (diluted formulation) (default for pyrethroids, 10%; for others, see section 4.1.2)

BW = body weight (adults 62 kg, older children 32 kg, toddlers 14 kg)

AT = averaging time, 1 year (365 days)

Ingestion via hand-to-mouth activity in toddlers can be calculated as previously described for residual disinsection.

If necessary, acute systemic doses can also be calculated using the same equations but omitting the terms for exposure frequency (EF) and averaging time (*AT*).

4.2.6 Total exposure assessment

The total exposure is calculated by summing the contribution of different exposure routes for all the appropriate scenarios relevant to a particular subgroup.

For estimation of the maximal daily exposure, to be compared with a guidance value for short-term exposure, the same algorithms can be used if the terms for exposure frequency (EF) and averaging time (AT) are omitted.

Table 5 provides a summary of aircraft disinsection procedures and the related exposures covered by this document.

4.2.7 Uncertainties and assumptions in exposure determining factors and risk calculations

Each of the default values represents a source of uncertainty. Some default values vary widely, depending on the source of data. For example, agricultural exposure databases seem to give higher estimates than databases relating to residential exposure. For some tasks, such as mixing and loading, the agricultural databases are more suitable as the tasks are similar in agricultural and public health settings. For application tasks, however, agricultural databases may not be the best sources.

The diversity of surface materials used makes it very difficult to estimate the persistence and decay of active ingredients on these surfaces. Also, the ease with which they are dislodged from surfaces is very difficult to estimate. Details of the decomposition of active ingredients – which is chemical-specific – are often unavailable. Assessing one-day acute dermal exposure to liquid formulations is assumed to give a conservative estimate of exposure.

Table 5. Disinsection procedures and related exposures

Procedures	Target groups	Exposure routes (direct[a])	Exposure routes (indirect[b])	Notes
Residual spraying before flight	Ground operators performing residual spraying	Inhalation, dermal		In some cases the cabin crew and the passengers are exposed both to residues of before-flight treatment *and* to space spray during flight. The exposures must then be summed up when appropriate (i.e. same active ingredient)
	In-flight personnel i.e. cabin crew		Dermal	
	Adult passengers		Dermal	
	Children		Dermal	
	Toddlers		Dermal, oral	
Space spraying during flight	In-flight personnel, i.e. cabin crew	Inhalation, dermal	Dermal	
	Adult passengers	Inhalation, dermal	Dermal	
	Children	Inhalation, dermal	Dermal	
	Toddlers	Inhalation, dermal	Dermal, oral	
	Infants	Inhalation		

[a] Direct exposure to insecticide from mixing and/or application/spraying.

[b] Indirect exposure via treated surfaces.

Default values used in the risk assessment models are often obtained from sources that relate to North American or European situations, which differ in many respects – for example, body dimensions – from African and Asian circumstances. In such cases, the use of conservative assumptions is most important. For body weight, the use of lower weights is the conservative approach since exposure is divided by body weight to obtain the systemic dose.

4.3 Risk characterization

The aim of risk characterization is to evaluate the probability of adverse effects occurring under defined exposure conditions. In its simplest form, risk characterization consists of the comparison of estimates of exposure with TSDs established in hazard assessment for all relevant exposure situations. Different TSDs are used for long-term and short-term exposure; these are typically derived from the ADI and the ARfD values, respectively, set by JMPR.

For long-term exposure, the comparison is defined as follows:

$$\text{Ratio} = \frac{\text{Estimated TWA systemic dose}}{\text{TSD}}$$

When the insecticide has significant acute toxicity (e.g. JMPR or another organization has established an ARfD), the risk is also estimated for short-term exposure compared with a short-term guidance value (TSD_{AC}):

$$\text{Ratio} = \frac{\text{Estimated maximal daily systemic dose}}{\text{TSD}_{\text{AC}}}$$

When these ratios are <1, the health risk is considered to be acceptable. When one or both are >1, there are possible health risks, and the planned use for aircraft disinsection may not be acceptable. In the case of operators, however, it may be possible to reduce the risk – for example by changing recommended operational conditions. A risk–benefit analysis, in which the risks of potential toxicity are compared with potential health benefits (disease prevention), may be needed in some cases.

The outcome of the risk characterization, the defaults used and any decisions taken should be clearly stated and justified.

5. CONCLUSIONS

The models described in this document are intended for first-tier risk assessments; if any better-validated models are available, they should be used. The default values presented here are meant to serve as examples; case- or substance-specific defaults or distributions for default parameters should be applied whenever available. In the interests of transparency of the process, it is of the utmost importance that the decisions taken are soundly and scientifically justified and accurately recorded.

6. SUMMARY OF THE HUMAN HEALTH RISK ASSESSMENT MODEL AND WORKED EXAMPLES

A summary of the risk assessment model together with worked examples is presented in this section. The active ingredient used as a model compound for each product is a pyrethroid insecticide.

Example exposure assessments are shown for two product types:

- a residual product supplied as an emulsifiable concentrate formulation (a 40% concentrate that is diluted with water to give a spray solution containing 2% active ingredient); and
- an aerosol spray can product, containing 2% active ingredient, to be used for space spraying within the aircraft cabin.

Generic risk assessment model	Worked example: pyrethroid insecticide "X"
1. Toxicity data	**1. Toxicity data**
Aim: To assess available toxicity data and derive acceptable exposure levels	*Aim:* To assess available toxicity data and derive acceptable exposure levels
1.1 Conduct literature search for human, animal and in-vitro toxicity data and any necessary physicochemical data on the insecticide	1.1 Literature search on insecticide "X" conducted on MEDLINE, TOXLINE and sources of reviews (WHO, IPCS, JMPR, USEPA, PSD, IARC, ATSDR, EFSA, etc.)
1.2 Obtain relevant reviews and key original papers	1.2 Comprehensive reviews available from IPCS, JMPR and IARC. Key original papers obtained.
1.3 Tabulate types of study, toxic effects observed, NOAELs and LOAELs	1.3 All available relevant animal and human studies tabulated
1.4 Assess whether quality of database is adequate for risk assessment (range of studies, conduct of studies, adequacy of dose–response data, etc.)	1.4 Studies available on all relevant types of toxicity, most via oral route, with some inhalation and dermal studies. Most conducted to acceptable standards with adequate dose–response data.

Generic risk assessment model	Worked example: pyrethroid insecticide "X"
1.5 If database is adequate, identify critical toxic effect(s)	1.5 In humans, first symptom of exposure is facial paraesthesia, reversible on cessation of exposure. Critical toxic effect in animal tests is neurotoxicity. No dose – response data are available for humans but database from animals is adequate.
1.6 If the insecticide is a skin or respiratory sensitizer, is genotoxic, carcinogenic or extremely acutely toxic, consider whether it is worth proceeding with risk assessment. Consider this also if the insecticide produces clear reproductive toxic effects at dose levels causing no general toxicity.	1.6 The substance is not genotoxic, and has not shown carcinogenic or specific reproductive toxic effects. Skin sensitization tests have been negative and no cases of skin or respiratory tract sensitization are reported in the scientific literature despite previous use of the insecticide in different applications. The substance has moderate acute toxicity. Toxicokinetic data suggests good oral absorption. Default 100% oral absorption is used in this assessment. Proceed with risk assessment.
1.7 If 1.6 does not apply, identify pivotal study/studies giving dose – response data for critical effect(s)	1.7 Pivotal studies are: – 21-day rat inhalation study – 1- and 2-year dog dietary studies – 2-year rat dietary study – acute rat oral neurotoxicity study
1.8 Identify critical NOAEL(s) from pivotal studies for acute exposure and for longer-term (repeat-dose) exposure	1.8 Critical NOAELs are: – 21-day inhalation (6 hours/day, 5 days/week), rat, NOAEC = 9.6 mg/m^3 (equivalent to 2.6 mg/kg bw per day) – 1- and 2-year dietary studies, dog, NOAEL = 1 mg/kg bw per day – 2-year rat dietary study, NOAEL= 1 mg/kg bw per day – acute rat neurotoxicity study, NOAEL = 5 mg/kg bw
1.9 Assess whether the database allows the setting of TSDs for short-term and long-term exposures.	1.9 Database adequate to allow setting of TSDs for single and repeated exposures

Generic risk assessment model	Worked example: pyrethroid insecticide "X"
1.10 Set TSDs for oral, dermal, or inhalation exposure by dividing NOAEL for the critical effect from the pivotal study via that route by an uncertainty factor (UF): TSD = NOAEL/UF (correcting for systemic bioavailability if necessary). A default UF of 100 is recommended for NOAELs derived from animal studies and 10 for NOAELs derived from human studies (see section 4.1.6 for variations on these defaults).	1.10 The ADI of 0.01 mg/kg bw per day is set by JMPR. This is based on 1- and 2-year dog studies and a 2-year rat study (all via the oral route), in which NOAELs of 1 mg/kg bw per day were identified. A subacute 21-day inhalation study with an NOAEL of 2.6 mg/kg bw per day supports these oral studies. Application of a UF of 100 to the lowest NOAEL, 1 mg/kg bw per day, results in a TSD of 0.01 mg/kg bw per day. Complete absorption from the gastrointestinal tract is indicated by the data, meaning that 0.01 mg/kg bw per day is considered to represent the tolerable systemic dose. JMPR has set also an ARfD of 0.05 mg/kg bw. This is based on a rat acute oral neurotoxicity study in which an NOAEL of 5 mg/kg bw was identified.
1.11 Conclusion on final TSD(s).	1.11 TSDs used in risk characterization: – long-term TSD, 0.01 mg/kg bw per day – short-term TSD_{AC}, 0.05 mg/kg bw

Generic risk assessment model	Worked example: residual product "X"
2. Exposure assessment: residual product "X" *Aim:* – to estimate occupational exposure via dermal and inhalation routes during mixing, loading and application of residual sprays in an aircraft for disinsection purposes; – to estimate exposure of adult and child passengers (post-application inhalation and dermal exposure, and toddlers' hand-to-mouth exposure).	**2. Exposure assessment: residual product "X"** An emulsifiable concentrate formulation of a pyrethroid insecticide, product "X", is to be used for residual spraying. The default dermal absorption value of 10% for pyrethroids applies. The guideline scenarios represent a situation in which label instructions are followed. In the lax standard scenarios, it may be assumed, for example, that no gloves are used or that spraying equipment is not totally leakproof.

Generic risk assessment model	Worked example: residual product "X"
The defaults and other data used in the assessments should not be limited to those presented as examples in this document. Searches should be made for case-specific, valid and scientifically sound data. Default values for absorption via the oral, dermal and inhalation routes are available if chemical-specific data are unavailable. Protection factor of adequate protective equipment, including gloves, is assumed to be 90%. Body weight is 62 kg for adults, 32 kg for older children and 14 kg for toddlers.	
2.1 Ground crew operator exposure *a) Mixing and loading* In mixing and loading, only dermal exposure is considered significant. It is assumed that the amount of the spray liquid prepared per day is three 10-litre tanks (sufficient to treat a large aircraft). It is also assumed that ground personnel treating the aircraft need to spray an aeroplane twice a week throughout the year.	***2.1 Ground crew operator exposure*** *a) Mixing and loading* Product used is a 40% emulsifiable concentrate formulation, supplied in 1-litre containers. The spray solution contains 2% of the active ingredient, prepared as 2 parts of the concentrate in 38 parts of distilled water. Chronic systemic dose due to dermal exposure, mg a.i./kg bw per day: 0.03 ml × 400 mg a.i./ml × 1.0 × 10% × 104 days/(62 kg × 365 days) **= 0.0055 mg a.i./kg bw per day** (lax standard scenario)

Generic risk assessment model	Worked example: residual product "X"
In the lax standard scenario, no gloves are assumed. In the guideline scenario, gloves are used. Default values for hand contamination per operation while mixing and loading are available in Table 4.	In the guideline scenario calculation, a protection factor of 90% applies, hence the systemic dose is: 0.03 ml × 400 mg a.i./ml × 0.1 × 10% × 104 days/(62 kg × 365 days) **= 0.00055 mg a.i./kg bw/day** The maximum daily systemic dose will be: 0.03 ml × 400 mg a.i./ml × 1.0 × 10%/62 kg **= 0.019 mg/kg bw** (lax standard scenario) 0.03 ml × 400 mg a.i./ml × 0.1 × 10%/62 kg **= 0.0019 mg/kg bw** (guideline scenario)
b) Application The quantity of spray to be applied depends on the area of the internal surfaces of the aircraft. The quantity to be used for different types of aircraft will be specified by the procedures of the national authority or by the product manufacturer. To calculate exposure it is necessary to know the target concentration of a.i. to be applied to the surfaces (mg/m^2) and the concentration of a.i. in the spray solution (mg/ml). For the area to be treated, a large aircraft is used for the example calculation. It is assumed, that 9.3 ml of spray liquid will contaminate the hands during one work day. Breathing rate 1.9 m^3/hour, work time 2 hours – air volume inhaled = 3.8 m^3.	*b) Application* The required dosage of the example product "X" is 200 mg/m^2. For the area and volume of the aircraft being treated, a large aircraft is assumed, with a surface area of 2500 m^2 and a volume of 1000 m^3. As the liquid being sprayed is a 2% emulsion, the spray concentration will be 20 mg/ml. The default absorption rate from the respiratory tract is 100%. Systemic dose due to inhalation exposure, mg a.i./kg bw per day: 200 mg/m^2 × 2500 m^2 × 0.001 × 1.0 × 3.8 m^3 × 100% × 104 days/(1000 m^3 × 62 kg × 365 days) = **0.0087 mg a.i./kg bw per day** (lax standard scenario) In the guideline scenario, the use of protective equipment provides a 90% protection factor. The exposure will therefore be 10% of that in the lax standard scenario, i.e. **0.00087 mg a.i./kg bw per day** The maximum daily systemic dose will be: 200 mg/m^2 × 2500 m^2 × 0.001 × 1.0 × 3.8 m^3 × 100%/(1000 m^3 × 62 kg) = **0.031 mg a.i./kg bw** (lax standard scenario) 200 mg/m^2 × 2500 m^2 × 0.001 × 0.1 × 3.8 m^3 × 100%/(1000 m^3 × 62 kg) = **0.0031 mg a.i./kg bw** (guideline scenario)

Generic risk assessment model	Worked example: residual product "X"
It is assumed that 0.1% of the a.i. sprayed will be evenly distributed in the air (including in the breathing zone of the operator).	Systemic dose due to dermal exposure, mg a.i./kg bw per day: 9.3 ml/day × 20 mg/ml × 1.0 × 10% × 104 days/(62 kg × 365 days) = **0.085 mg a.i./kg bw per day** (lax standard scenario) In the guideline scenario calculation, the protection factor for protective clothing (90%) is applied, and the systemic dose is **0.0085 mg a.i./kg bw per day** The maximum daily systemic dose will be: 9.3 ml/day × 20 mg/ml × 1.0 × 10%/62 kg = **0.3 mg a.i./kg bw** (lax standard scenario) 9.3 ml/day × 20 mg/ml × 0.1 × 10%/62 kg = **0.03 mg a.i./kg bw** (guideline scenario)
2.2 Cabin crew and passenger exposure from residual disinsection Passenger and cabin crew exposure is assumed to be due to secondary dermal exposure from contact with the surfaces of the aircraft. For passengers and cabin crew, the proportion translodged onto bare skin is 11%; the exposed area of skin reflects the clothing worn, with an additional component for toddlers because of greater activity. For cabin crew, the exposed skin area is 0.1 m^2 (50% of hands and forearms) and the exposure duration is 240 days per year.	***2.2 Cabin crew and passenger exposure from residual disinsection*** Product-specific target concentration on the surfaces, 0.2 g/m^2 = 200 mg/m^2 Systemic dose of cabin crew members due to dermal exposure, mg a.i./kg bw per day: 200 mg/m^2 × 11% × 0.1 m^2 × 10% × 240 days/(62 kg × 365 days) = **0.002 mg a.i./kg bw per day** Maximum daily exposure: 200 mg/m^2 × 11% × 0.1 m^2 × 10%/ 62 kg = **0.0035 mg a.i./kg bw** Systemic dose of the passengers due to dermal exposure, mg a.i./kg bw per day: 200 mg/m^2 × 11% × (0.25 m^2, 0.16 m^2 or 0.2 m^2) × 10% × (40 days or 5 days)/((62 kg, 32 kg or 14 kg) × 365 days) Long-term exposures: for adults: **0.00097 mg a.i./kg bw per day** for children: **0.00015 mg a.i./kg bw per day** for toddlers: **0.00043 mg a.i./kg bw per day**

Generic risk assessment model	Worked example: residual product "X"
For passengers, the exposed skin areas are 0.25 m^2 for adults, 0.16 m^2 for older children, and 0.2 m^2 for toddlers. Exposure duration is 40 days for adult passengers and 5 days for children. In addition, the sprayed insecticide may be dislodged from surfaces as contaminated dust leading to ingestion by toddlers due to hand-to-mouth behaviour. For estimating the hand-to-mouth exposure, the relevant hand area for toddlers is 0.032 m^2. For the extent of the transfer from hands to mouth, a default of 10% is used.	Maximum daily exposures: for adults: **0.0088 mg a.i./kg bw** for children: **0.011 mg a.i./kg bw** for toddlers: **0.031 mg a.i./kg bw** Systemic dose due to hand-to-mouth behaviour, toddlers, mg a.i./kg bw per day: 200 mg/m^2 × 11% × 0.032 m^2 × 10% × 100% × 5 days/(14 kg × 365 days) = **0.00007 mg a.i./kg bw per day** Maximum daily exposure: 200 mg/m^2 × 11% × 0.032 m^2 × 10% × 100%/14 kg = **0.005 mg a.i./kg bw**
3. Risk characterization	**3. Risk characterization**
3.1 Compare exposure estimates with TSDs for risk characterization. For products with appreciable acute toxicity, comparison against TSD_{AC} should also be considered. 3.2 If the exposure calculated for a subgroup and exposure route is below the respective TSD, using conservative estimates, it can be assumed that the exposure is acceptable and does not cause unacceptable risk to human health.	Insecticide "X" has moderate acute toxicity. Thus the risk assessment is based on: – comparison of chronic exposure with the long-term TSD; – comparison of acute exposure with the short-term TSD_{AC}. From section 1.10 of this worked example, the TSD used in long-term risk characterization is 0.01 mg/kg bw per day. Short-term guidance value (TSD_{AC}) is 0.05 mg/kg bw per day. ***Predicted doses to be used in subsequent risk characterization*** *Total operator predicted dose, ground personnel performing residual disinsections:* • Long-term (TWA) exposure

Generic risk assessment model	Worked example: residual product "X"
3.3 If the exposure is above the TSD and refining the assessment process, e.g. by use of chemical-specific data, fails to bring the exposure below the TSD, measures to reduce the exposure must be implemented. 3.4 In some cases the exposure may be found to be unacceptable despite measures to reduce it. Other methods of vector control should be considered.	Lax standard scenario: $dose_{M/L}$ dermal + $dose_A$ inhalation + $dose_A$ dermal = 0.0055 + 0.0087 + 0.085 **= 0.099 mg a.i./kg bw per day** Guideline scenario: $dose_{M/L}$ dermal + $dose_A$ $dose_{M/L}$ dermal + $dose_A$ inhalation + $dose_A$ dermal = 0.00055 + 0.00087 + 0.0085 **= 0.0099 mg a.i./kg bw per day** where: $dose_{M/L}$ refers to exposure from mixing and loading, and $dose_A$ refers to exposure from application In the guideline exposure scenario, worker exposure is considered to be acceptable, as the total predicted dose is similar to the TSD. In the lax standard scenario, the TSD may be exceeded by a factor of 10. It is therefore important to ensure that safe practices are implemented, that adequate PPE is used and that the equipment is maintained in good working condition. • Acute (maximal daily) exposure Lax standard scenario: $dose_{M/L}$ dermal + $dose_A$ inhalation + $dose_A$ dermal = 0.019 + 0.031 + 0.3 = **0.35 mg a.i./kg bw** Guideline scenario: $dose_{M/L}$ dermal + $dose_A$ inhalation + $dose_A$ dermal = 0.0019 + 0.0031 + 0.03 = **0.035 mg a.i./kg bw**

Generic risk assessment model	Worked example: residual product "X"
	In the guideline exposure scenario, acute worker exposure is considered to be acceptable, as the maximal daily dose is approximately 70% of the TSD_{AC}. In the lax standard scenario, the TSD_{AC} may be exceeded by a factor of 7. It is therefore important to ensure that safe practices are implemented, that adequate PPE is used and that the equipment is maintained in good working condition. *Total cabin crew predicted dose:* Dose from touching contaminated surfaces = **0.002 mg a.i./kg bw per day (TWA) or 0.0035 mg a.i./kg bw (maximal daily exposure)** Cabin crew exposure is considered to be acceptable. The predicted doses are 23% of the TSD and 7% of the TSD_{AC}. *Total passenger predicted doses:* • Long-term exposure: for adult passengers **0.00097 mg a.i./kg bw per day** for children **0.00015 mg a.i./kg bw per day** • Maximum daily exposures: for adult passengers **0.0088 mg a.i./kg bw** for children **0.011 mg a.i./kg bw** Exposure of adult and child passengers from residual treatment is considered to be acceptable - the predicted doses are less than 10% of the TSD and less than 22% of the TSD_{AC}.

Generic risk assessment model	Worked example: residual product "X"
	Total passenger predicted doses – toddlers: • Long-term dose from touching contaminated surfaces + dose from hand-to-mouth behaviour = 0.00043 + 0.00007 = **0.0005 mg a.i./kg bw per day** • Maximum daily exposure from touching contaminated surfaces + dose from hand-to-mouth behaviour = 0.031 + 0.005 = **0.036 mg a.i./kg bw** Exposure of toddlers from residual treatment is considered to be acceptable – the predicted doses represent 5% and 73% of the TSD and TSD_{AC}, respectively.

Generic risk assessment model	Worked example: aerosol spray product "X"
4. Exposure assessment *Aim:* – to estimate occupational exposure via dermal and inhalation routes resulting from spraying aerosol sprays in an aircraft for disinsection purposes; – to estimate exposure of adult and child passengers (post-application inhalation and dermal exposure). The defaults and other data used in the assessments should not be limited to those presented as examples in this document. Searches should be made for case-specific, valid and scientifically sound data.	**4. Exposure assessment: aerosol product "X"** In this worked example, the product is an aerosol can containing 2% of the pyrethroid active ingredient with a propellant approved for use in aircraft. The default dermal absorption value of 10% for pyrethroids applies. As an example, a large aircraft is used (cabin volume 1000 m^3). As the required coverage of the formulation is 35 g /100 m^3, or 350 mg/m^3), a total of 4 × 100 gram cans should be completely emptied during this procedure.

Generic risk assessment model	Worked example: aerosol spray product “X”
Default values for absorption via the dermal and inhalation routes are available if chemical-specific data are not available. Body weight is 62 kg for adults, 32 kg for older children and 14 kg for toddlers. Body weight for newborn infants (exposed via inhalation only) is 4.8 kg.	
4.1 Space spraying, cabin crew exposure, application Default values for the general exposure parameters needed for inhalation exposure assessment with ConsExpo software are: – the spray duration (in this case estimated 200 seconds); – exposure duration (30 minutes); – room volume (or in this case, volume of the cabin, large aircraft, default 1000 m^3); – room height (estimated 2 m); – ventilation rate (as a worst case it is assumed that there is no effect due to ventilation).	***4.1 Space spraying, cabin crew exposure, application*** The product specific parameters required by the ConsExpo inhalation model are: – the mass generation rate, or the amount of compound released from the can during spraying per unit of time (2 g/s to reflect the number of cans being discharged simultaneously in this example scenario); – estimate of the airborne, non-volatile fraction (a worst-case assumption has been made, that this fraction is 100%); – inhalation cut-off droplet diameter (15 μm); – weight fraction of non-volatiles (default 2%); – weight fraction of compound of interest in the product (percentage of a.i. in the product, 2%); – density of non-volatile compounds (assumed 1.8 g/cm^3); – initial particle distribution (assumed log-normal, average particle diameter 8 μm, coefficient of variation 0.45).

Generic risk assessment model	Worked example: aerosol spray product "X"
The remaining parameters needed for the software are product-specific. Respiration rate of cabin crew members is assumed to be 0.89 m^3/h. Space spray is not intended to settle on surfaces, but is likely to be carried away by the air circulation. It can be assumed that 1% of the material sprayed into the air could be deposited on the surfaces. A large aircraft with a volume of 1000 m^3 and an internal surface area (including internal fittings) of 2500 m^2 is assumed. The guideline scenarios represent a situation in which label instructions are being followed and assume that the products used are in good working condition. Touching surfaces is the only source of dermal exposure in the guideline scenario. In the lax standard scenarios, it may be assumed, for example, that the spray nozzle may leak onto the fingers; no gloves are used.	The amount of material sprayed into the air for this product is calculated as: 200 seconds × 2 g/s of product = 400 g product (containing 8 g of active ingredient). Of this, 1% could be deposited on surfaces – 1% of 8 g divided by an internal surface area of 2500 m^2 = 0.032 mg/m^2. *Systemic dose due to inhalation exposure:* These exposure estimates are obtained directly from the output of the ConsExpo software. The algorithms behind the ConsExpo spray model are not shown in this worked example – they are readily available from the Internet. **0.012 mg a.i./kg bw per day** (ConsExpo Output – inhalation chronic systemic dose, point-estimate) **0.019 mg a.i./kg bw per day** (ConsExpo Output – inhalation acute systemic dose, point-estimate) *Systemic dose due to dermal exposure via body areas in contact with surfaces:* 0.032 mg/m^2 × 11% × 0.1 m^2 × 240 days × 10%/62 kg × 365 days = **0.000 000 4 mg a.i./kg bw per day** *Systemic dose due to dermal exposure via contamination of fingers with spray liquid (leaking nozzle):* 1 ml/day × 20 mg/ml × 240 days × 10%/62 kg × 365 days = **0.02 mg a.i./kg bw per day** For guideline scenario, systemic dose due to dermal exposure = contact with surfaces only = **0.000 000 4 mg a.i./kg bw per day** For lax standard scenario, systemic dose due to dermal exposure = contact with surfaces + contamination of fingers = 0.000 000 4 + 0.02 = **0.02 mg a.i./kg bw per day**

Generic risk assessment model	Worked example: aerosol spray product "X"
	• Maximum daily exposures from body areas in contact with surfaces: 0.032 mg/m^2 × 11% × 0.1 m^2 × 10%/62 kg = **0.000 000 6 mg a.i./kg bw** • Maximum daily exposures from contamination of fingers: 1 ml/day × 20 mg/ml × 10%/62 kg = **0.032 mg a.i./kg bw** For guideline scenario, maximum daily dermal exposure is: **0.000 000 6 mg a.i./kg bw** For lax standard scenario, maximum daily dermal exposure is: 0.000 000 6 + 0.032 = **0.032 mg a.i./kg bw**
4.2 Space spraying, passenger exposure For the systemic dose due to indirect dermal exposure (to material deposited on surfaces), exposed skin areas are 0.25 m^2 for adults, 0.16 m^2 for older children, 0.2 m^2 for toddlers. The material deposited on surfaces is calculated in the same way as for cabin crew. If passengers are present during space spraying, the pattern of inhalation exposure is considered to be similar to crew members' exposure. Exposure frequencies are 40 days/year for adult passengers and 5 days/year for children of	***4.2 Space spraying, passenger exposure*** *Systemic dose due to indirect dermal exposure (passengers not present during space spraying – body areas in contact with surfaces where material has deposited)*: 0.032 mg/m^2 × 11% × (0.25, 0.16 or 0.2 m^2) × (40 or 5 days) × 10%/(62, 32 or 14 kg) × 365 days (chronic exposure) for adult passengers **0.000 000 2 mg a.i./kg bw per day** for children **0.000 000 02 mg a.i./kg bw per day** for toddlers **0.000 000 07 mg a.i./kg bw per day** • Maximal daily exposure 0.032 mg/m^2 × 11% × (0.25, 0.16 or 0.2m^2) × 10%/(62, 32 or 14 kg) for adult passengers **0.000 001 4 mg a.i./kg bw**

Generic risk assessment model	Worked example: aerosol spray product "X"
all ages. See model parameters used in cabin crew exposure calculations. Breathing rates (resting rates) for adult passengers are 0.40 m^3/h, for children 6–11 years and toddlers 0.38 m^3/h, and for newborn infants 0.28 m^3/h. For the systemic dose due to direct dermal contact with the spray, exposed skin areas are 0.33 m^2 for adults, 0.26 m^2 for older children, and 0.15 m^2 for toddlers (based on the head and half of the hands, forearms and lower legs). For newborn infants, only inhalation exposure is considered to be relevant because infants will be held or transported in their own carriers and will have very limited opportunity for contact with aircraft surfaces.	for children **0.000 001 8 mg a.i./kg bw** for toddlers **0.000 005 mg a.i./kg bw** *Systemic dose due to inhalation exposure (passengers present during space spraying):* The exposure estimates are obtained directly from the output of the ConsExpo software. The underlying algorithms are not shown in this worked example: for adult passengers **0.000 93 mg a.i./kg bw per day (chronic)** **0.0085 mg a.i./kg bw (acute)** for children **0.000 21 mg a.i./kg bw per day (chronic)** **0.016 mg a.i./kg bw (acute)** for toddlers **0.000 51 mg a.i./kg bw per day (chronic)** **0.038 mg a.i./kg bw (acute)** for newborn infants **0.0011 mg a.i./kg bw per day (chronic)** **0.077 mg a.i./kg bw (acute)** (ConsExpo Output – inhalation systemic doses, point-estimates) *Systemic dose due to direct skin contact with the spray (passengers present during space spraying:* 0.032 mg/m^2 × (0.33, 0.26 or 0.15 m^2) × (40 or 5 days) × 10%/(62, 32 or 14 kg) × 365 days (chronic exposure) for adult passengers **0.000 002 mg a.i./kg bw per day** for children **0.000 000 4 mg a.i./kg bw per day** for toddlers **0.000 000 5 mg a.i./kg bw per day**

Generic risk assessment model	Worked example: aerosol spray product "X"
	• Maximal daily exposure $0.032\ mg/m^2 \times (0.33, 0.26$ or $0.15\ m^2) \times 10\%/(62, 32$ or $14\ kg)$ for adult passengers **0.000 017 mg a.i./kg bw** for children **0.000 026 mg a.i./kg bw** for toddlers **0.000 034 mg a.i./kg bw**
5. Risk characterization	**5. Risk characterization**
5.1 Compare exposure estimates with TSDs for risk characterization. For products with appreciable acute toxicity, consideration should be given to comparing against TSD_{AC}.	Insecticide "X" has moderate acute toxicity. Thus the risk assessment is based on: – comparison of chronic exposure with the long-term TSD; – comparison of acute exposure with the short-term TSD_{AC}.
5.2 If the exposure calculated for a subgroup and exposure route is below the respective TSD, using conservative estimates, it can be assumed that the exposure is acceptable and does not cause unacceptable risk to human health. 5.3 If the exposure is above the TSD and refining the assessment process, e.g. by use of chemical-specific data, fails to bring the exposure below the TSD, measures to reduce the exposure must be implemented.	From section 1.10 of this worked example, the TSD used in long-term risk characterization is 0.01 mg/kg bw per day. Short-term guidance value (TSD_{AC}) is 0.05 mg/kg bw per day. ***Predicted doses to be used in subsequent risk characterization:*** *Total predicted dose, cabin crew performing space spraying:* • Long-term (TWA) exposure Lax standard scenario: $Inhalation_{dose}$ + Dermal contact with $surfaces_{dose}$ + Contamination of $fingers_{dose}$ = 0.012 + 0.000 000 4 + 0.02 = **0.032 mg a.i./kg bw per day** Guideline scenario: $Inhalation_{dose}$ + Dermal contact with $surfaces_{dose}$ = 0.012 + 0.000 000 4 = **0.012 mg a.i./kg bw/day**

Generic risk assessment model	Worked example: aerosol spray product "X"
5.4 In some cases the exposure may be found to be unacceptable despite measures to reduce it. Other methods of vector control should ben considered.	In the guideline exposure scenario, the exposure is approximately equal to the TSD. The fact that the models tend to use conservative estimates needs to be taken into account when evaluating the significance of exposures that are close to the TSD (for example, in this scenario no effect of ventilation is assumed). In the lax standard scenario, the predicted exposure exceeds the TSD by a factor of 3. Most of the exposure in this scenario results from contamination of the fingers due to leaking spray nozzles – which should occur very rarely in practice and represents a very conservative estimate. However, this estimate shows that it is essential that the products used are in good working condition. Since this lower-tier exposure estimate exceeds the health-based guidance value, higher-tier estimates of exposure should be considered. For example – models for the contamination of the hands while using an aerosol spray can are available within ConsExpo. • Acute (maximal daily) exposure Lax standard scenario: $Inhalation_{dose}$ + Dermal contact with $surfaces_{dose}$ + Contamination of $fingers_{dose}$ = 0.019 + 0.000 000 6 + 0.032 = **0.051 mg a.i./kg bw** Guideline scenario: $Inhalation_{dose}$ + Dermal contact with $surfaces_{dose}$ = 0.019 + 0.000 000 6 = **0.019 mg a.i./kg bw**

Generic risk assessment model	Worked example: aerosol spray product "X"
	In the guideline exposure scenario, the exposure is considered acceptable as the predicted exposure is 38% of the TSD_{AC}. In the lax standard scenario the exposure is approximately equal to the TSD_{AC}. *Predicted doses for passengers from indirect exposure* In this scenario passengers were not present when spraying was carried out and they are exposed through touching surfaces contaminated with spray deposit (in contrast to residual spraying where the deposit on surfaces is intentional): for adult passengers **0.000 000 2 mg a.i./kg bw per day (chronic)** **0.000 001 4 mg a.i./kg bw (acute)** for children **0.000 000 02 mg a.i./kg bw per day (chronic)** **0.000 001 8 mg a.i./kg bw (acute)** for toddlers **0.000 000 07 mg a.i./kg bw per day (chronic)** **0.000 005 mg a.i./kg bw (acute)** In all cases these exposures are considered to be acceptable because the predicted doses are well below the TSD or TSD_{AC} (<1%). *Predicted doses for passengers from direct exposure* In this scenario passengers are present when spraying is carried out and they are exposed through inhalation and also through direct skin contact with the spray while spraying is taking place: for adult passengers $Inhalation_{dose}$ + Skin contact with $spray_{dose}$ = 0.000 93 + 0.000 002 = **0.000 93 mg a.i./kg bw per day (chronic)**

<table>
<tr><th>Generic risk assessment model</th><th>Worked example: aerosol spray product "X"</th></tr>
<tr><td></td><td>This is 9% of the TSD.
$Inhalation_{dose}$ + Skin contact with $spray_{dose}$
= 0.008 5 + 0.000 017
= 0.008 5 mg a.i./kg bw (acute)
This is 17% of the TSD_{AC}.
for children
$Inhalation_{dose}$ + Skin contact with $spray_{dose}$
= 0.000 21 + 0.000 000 4
= 0.000 21 mg a.i./kg bw per day (chronic)
This is 2% of the TSD.
$Inhalation_{dose}$ + Skin contact with $spray_{dose}$
= 0.016 + 0.000 026
= 0.016 mg a.i./kg bw (acute)
This is 32% of the TSD_{AC}.
for toddlers
$Inhalation_{dose}$ + Skin contact with $spray_{dose}$
= 0.000 51 + 0.000 000 5
= 0.000 51 mg a.i./kg bw per day (chronic)
This is 5% of the TSD.
$Inhalation_{dose}$ + Skin contact with $spray_{dose}$
= 0.038 + 0.000 034
= 0.038 mg a.i./kg bw (acute)
This is 76% of the TSD_{AC}.
The exposures for adults, older children and toddlers in this scenario are considered to be acceptable because the predicted doses are below the TSD or TSD_{AC} in all cases.
For this scenario, where passengers are present when spraying is carried out, it is also necessary to consider the exposure of newborn infants via inhalation.
For infants
$Inhalation_{dose}$
= 0.0011 mg a.i./kg bw per day (chronic)
= 0.077 mg a.i./kg bw (acute)</td></tr>
</table>

Generic risk assessment model	Worked example: aerosol spray product "X"
	Exposure of newborn infants is considered to be acceptable on a chronic basis as the predicted dose is 11% of the TSD. For acute exposure, the TSD_{AC} is exceeded (154%). Higher-tier assessment should be considered, taking into account the conservative assumptions used in this initial assessment (for example the initial assessment assumes no effect due to ventilation).

REFERENCES

Berger-Preiss E et al. (2004). In-flight spraying in aircrafts: determination of the exposure scenario. *International Journal of Hygiene and Environmental Health*, **207**: 419–430.

Berger-Preiss E et al. (2006). Aircraft disinsection: exposure assessment and evaluation of a new pre-embarkation method. *International Journal of Hygiene and Environmental Health*, **209**: 41–56.

Bremmer HJ, Prud'Homme de Lodder LCH, van Engelen JGM (2006). *General Fact Sheet – Limiting conditions and reliability, ventilation, room size, body surface area*, updated version for ConsExpo 4. Bilthoven, National Institute for Public Health and the Environment (RIVM Report 320104002, available at: http://www.rivm.nl/dsresource?objectid=rivmp:13091&type=org&disposition=inline).

CRD (2007). *UK Predictive Operator Exposure Model (POEM)*. York, Chemicals Regulation Directorate (available at: http://www.pesticides.gov.uk/approvals.asp?id=2427).

DAFF/MPI (2012). *Schedule of aircraft disinsection procedures for flights into Australia and New Zealand. Version 2.2*. Canberra, Department of Agriculture, Fisheries and Forestry, and Wellington, Ministry for Primary Industries (available at: http://www.daff.gov.au/biosecurity/avm/aircraft/disinsection/procedures).

Delmaar JE, Park MVDZ, van Engelen JGM (2005). *ConsExpo 4.0. Consumer exposure and uptake models: program manual*. Bilthoven, National Institute for Public Health and the Environment (RIVM report 320104004/2005; available at: http://www.rivm.nl/en/healthanddisease/productsafety/ConsExpo.jsp#Software_model_to_calculate_consumer_exposure).

Delmaar JE, Bremmer HJ (2009). *The ConsExpo spray model. Modelling and experimental validation of the inhalation exposure of consumers to aerosols from spray cans and trigger sprays*. Bilthoven, National Institute for Public Health and the Environment (RIVM Report RIVM Report 320104005/2009; available at: http://www.rivm.nl/en/Library/Scientific/Reports/2010/januari/The_ConsExpo_spray_model_Modelling_and_experimental_validation_of_the_inhalation_exposure_of_consumers_to_aerosols_from_spray_cans_and_trigger_sprays).

Dorne JL, Renwick AG (2005). The refinement of uncertainty/safety factors in risk assessment by the incorporation of data on toxicokinetic variability in humans. *Toxicological Sciences*, **86(1)**: 20–26.

Dourson ML, Knauf LA, Swartout JC (1992). On reference dose (RfD) and its underlying toxicity data base. *Toxicology and Industrial Health*, **8**: 171–189.

EC (2002). *Guidance document on dermal absorption.* Brussels, European Commission (SANCO/222/2000 rev 6, 27 November 2002).

EC (2006). *Draft guidance for the setting and application of acceptable operator exposure levels (AOELs): working document.* Brussels, European Commission (available at: http://ec.europa.eu/food/plant/protection/resources/7531_rev_10.pdf).

EUROPOEM II (2003). *The development, maintenance and dissemination of a European Predictive Operator Exposure Model (EUROPOEM) database. A EUROPOEM II Database and Harmonised Model, FAIR3-CT96-1406.* Carshalton, England, TNO-BIBRA International.

Herrman JL, Younes M (1999). Background to the ADI/TDI/PTWI. *Regulatory Toxicology and Pharmacology*, **30**: S109–S113.

HSL (2011). *Bayesian Exposure Assessment Toolkit (BEAT).* Buxton, England, Health & Safety Laboratory (available at: http://xnet.hsl.gov.uk/download/).

JMPM (2008). *Second Session of the FAO/WHO Joint Meeting on Pesticide Management and 4th Session of the FAO Panel of Experts on Pesticide Management, Geneva, 6–8 October 2008: Recommendations.* Rome, Food and Agriculture Organization of the United Nations (available at: http://www.fao.org/fileadmin/templates/agphome/documents/Pests_Pesticides/Code/ Recommendations08_01.pdf).

Llewellyn DM et al. (1996). Occupational exposure to permethrin during its use as a public hygiene insecticide. *Annals of Occupational Hygiene*, **40**: 499–509.

Matthews GA (2001). Dermal exposure of hands to pesticides. In: Maibach HI (ed.) Toxicology of skin. Philadelphia, PA, Taylor and Francis: 179–182.

Meek ME et al (2011). Risk assessment of combined exposure to multiple chemicals: A WHO/IPCS framework. *Regulatory Toxicology and Pharmacology*, **60**: S1–S14.

Najera JA, Zaim M (2001). *Malaria vector control – insecticides for indoor residual spraying.* Geneva, World Health Organization (WHO/CDS/WHOPES/2001.3).

OECD (1987). *Guidelines for the testing of chemicals* (and subsequent revisions). Paris, Organisation for Economic Cooperation and Development (available at:www.oecd.org/env/testguidelines).

Solecki R et al. (2005). Guidance on setting of acute reference dose (ARfD) for pesticides. *Food and Chemical Toxicology,* **43**: 1569–1593.

Solecki R et al. (2010). A retrospective analysis of acute reference doses for pesticides evaluated in the European Union. *Critical Reviews in Toxicology*, **40(1)**: 24–34.

Sutton PM et al. (2007). Pesticide illness among flight attendants due to aircraft disinsection. *American Journal of Industrial Medicine*, **50**: 345–356.

UNECE (2011). *Globally Harmonized System of Classification and Labelling of Chemicals (GHS)*. Geneva, United Nations Economic Commission for Europe (available at: http://www.unece.org/trans/danger/publi/ghs/ghs_welcome_e.html).

USEPA (1997a). *Standard operating procedures for residential exposure assessments.* Washington, DC, United States Environmental Protection Agency, Office of Science Coordination and Policy, USA (available at: www.epa.gov/oscpmont/sap/meetings/1997/september/sopindex.htm).

USEPA (1997b). *Exposure factors handbook.* Washington, DC, United States Environmental Protection Agency, National Center for Environmental Assessment (available at: http://cfpub.epa.gov/ncea/cfm/recordisplay.cfm?deid=12464).

USEPA (2008). *Child-specific exposure factors handbook (final report)*. Washington, DC, United States Environmental Protection Agency, Office of Research and Development (available at: http://cfpub.epa.gov/ncea/cfm/recordisplay.cfm?deid=199243).

USEPA (2009). *Standard operating procedures (SOPs) for residential pesticide exposure assessments. Draft Technical Guidelines.* Submitted to the FIFRA Scientific Advisory Panel for review and comment October 6–9, 2009. Washington DC, United States Environmental Protection Agency, Office of Pesticide Programs, Office of Prevention, Pesticides, and Toxic Substances.

USEPA (2011). *Exposure factors handbook: 2011 edition*. Washington, DC, United States Environmental Protection Agency, National Center for Environmental Assessment (available at: http://cfpub.epa.gov/ncea/cfm/recordisplay.cfm?deid=236252).

Vermeire T et al. (1999). Assessment factors for human health risk assessment: a discussion paper. *Critical Reviews in Toxicology*, **29**: 439–490.

WHO (1985). Recommendations on the disinsecting of aircraft. *Weekly Epidemiological Record*, **60(7)**: 45–47.

WHO (1994). *Assessing human health risks of chemicals: derivation of guidance values for health-based exposure limits*. Geneva, World Health Organization (Environmental Health Criteria, 170; available at: http://www.inchem.org/documents/ehc/ehc/ehc170.htm).

WHO (1995). *Report of the Informal Consultation on Aircraft Disinsection. WHO/HQ, Geneva, 6–10 November 1995*. Geneva, World Health Organization (WHO/PCS/95.51, available at: http://whqlibdoc.who.int/HQ/1995/WHO_PCS_95.51_Rev.pdf).

WHO (1999). *Principles for the assessment of risks to human health from exposure to chemicals*. Geneva, World Health Organization (Environmental Health Criteria, 210; available at: http://www.inchem.org/documents/ehc/ehc/ehc210.htm).

WHO (2003). *Space spray application of insecticides for vector and public health pest control – a practitioner's guide*. Geneva, World Health Organization (WHO/CDS/WHOPES/GCDPP/2003.5; available at: http://whqlibdoc.who.int/hq/2003/WHO_CDS_WHOPES_GCDPP_2003.5.pdf).

WHO (2005a). *International Health Regulations*, 2nd ed. Geneva, World Health Organization (available at: http://www.who.int/ihr/9789241596664/en/index.html).

WHO (2005b). *Safety of pyrethroids for public health use*. Geneva, World Health Organization, Geneva (WHO/CDS/WHOPES/GCDPP/2005.10; available at: http://whqlibdoc.who.int/hq/2005/WHO_CDS_WHOPES_GCDPP_2005.10.pdf).

WHO (2005c). *Chemical-specific adjustment factors for interspecies differences and human variability: guidance document for use of data in dose/concentration–response assessment*. Geneva, World Health Organization (IPCS Harmonization Project Document No. 2; available at: http://whqlibdoc.who.int/publications/2005/9241546786_eng.pdf).

WHO (2006). *Equipment for vector control – specification guidelines*. Geneva, World Health Organization (available at: http://www.who.int/whopes/equipment/en/).

WHO (2007). *Manual for indoor residual spraying: application of residual sprays for vector control*, 3rd ed. Geneva, World Health Organization (available at: http://whqlibdoc.who.int/HQ/2007/WHO_CDS_NTD_WHOPES_GCDPP_2007.3_eng.pdf).

WHO (2008). *Uncertainty and data quality in exposure assessment. Part 1: Guidance document on characterizing and communicating uncertainty in exposure assessment*. Geneva, World Health Organization (IPCS Harmonization Project Document No. 6; available at: http://whqlibdoc.who.int/publications/2008/9789241563765_eng.pdf).

WHO (2009). *Principles and methods for the risk assessment of chemicals in food*. Geneva, World Health Organization (Environmental Health Criteria, 240; available at: http://www.who.int/foodsafety/chem/principles/en/index1.html).

WHO (2010). *WHO recommended classification of pesticides by hazard and guidelines to classification*. Geneva, World Organization (available at: http://whqlibdoc.who.int/publications/2010/9789241547963_eng.pdf).

WHO (2011a). *Generic risk assessment model for indoor residual spraying of insecticides*, 1st revision. Geneva, World Health Organization

(WHO/HTM/NTD/WHOPES/2010.5.Rev1; available at: http://whqlibdoc.who.int/publications/2011/9789241502177_eng.pdf).

WHO (2011b). *Generic risk assessment model for indoor and outdoor space spraying of insecticides*, 1st revision. Geneva, World Health Organization (available at: http://whqlibdoc.who.int/publications/2011/9789241501682_eng.pdf

WHO (2012a). *Guidelines for testing the efficacy of insecticide products used in aircraft*. Geneva, World Health (available at: http://whqlibdoc.who.int/publications/2012/9789241503235_eng.pdf).

WHO (2012b). *A generic risk assessment model for insecticide-treated nets*, revised ed. Geneva, World Health (available at: http://whqlibdoc.who.int/publications/2012/9789241503419_eng.pdf).

PART B

EVALUATION OF CHEMICAL INSECTICIDE PRODUCTS INTENDED FOR USE IN AIRCRAFT DISINSECTION

INTRODUCTION

Part B presents evaluations of different types of aircraft disinsection products against the criteria specified in the "*Generic risk assessment model for disinsection of aircraft with chemical insecticides*" described in Part A of this publication.

In developing the risk assessment model it was necessary to identify the different types of product which are currently being used or developed, and the various exposure scenarios which needed to be covered.

Information on aircraft disinsection products which are available on the market now, or which are currently being developed, was provided to WHO on a voluntary basis by product manufacturers.

The information provided by the manufacturers was supplemented by toxicity data on the active ingredients from authoritative international assessments (JMPR and EFSA) in line with section 4.1 of the generic risk assessment model. These data were used to derive tolerable systemic dose levels and a dermal absorption value.

The evaluations of the different types of products against the criteria in the risk assessment model are presented to assist governmental organizations in WHO Member States when considering aircraft disinsection products within their jurisdiction.

The evaluations are presented according to the use of the various type of products.

The regulatory approval of products and methods for aircraft disinsection is the sole prerogative and responsibility of national authorities.

The evaluations presented in this publication do not represent or imply any endorsement, recommendation, approval or rejection by WHO of the type of products concerned.

The quality, efficacy and safety of any disinsection product may be adversely affected by improper storage, handling and transportation.

The evaluations in this publication only remain valid if products are stored, handled and transported as recommended by the product manufacturer.

The evaluations conducted by WHO are aimed solely at assessing the risk to human health of the type of products concerned. The evaluations did not include an assessment of efficacy and/or product quality. Guidance on the assessment of the efficacy and quality of insecticide products is published by the WHO Pesticide Evaluation Scheme (WHOPES), and can be found at www.who.int/whopes.

The evaluations presented in this publication are based on information available to WHO at the time the evaluations were conducted. WHO cannot represent that manufacturers of the types of product that were evaluated, will not subsequently make changes (for example, to the product formulation or to the recommended conditions of use) which could affect the outcome of the evaluation presented. WHO does not furthermore warrant or represent that the evaluations conducted by it are complete or error free.

The publication of these evaluations does not replace the need for national authorities to conduct their own evaluations (in regard to the risk to human health, efficacy and product quality). National authorities should ensure that regulatory decisions are based on complete up-to-date information regarding the product being evaluated.

The types of product which have been evaluated do not represent an exhaustive list of all of the types of product which could potentially be used in aircraft disinsection. WHO advises national authorities to assess the risk to human health of new types of product which are not evaluated in this publication, on the basis of the methodology presented in Part A.

This publication may not be used by manufacturers and distributors for commercial or promotional purposes. However, manufacturers are encouraged to evaluate their aircraft disinsection products using the methods and criteria presented in Part A of this publication when submitting applications for regulatory approval, provided always that manufacturers and distributors shall not be entitled to use the name, acronym and/or emblem of WHO.

EVALUATION OF RESIDUAL SPRAY CONCENTRATE PRODUCTS (PERMETHRIN)

Product type: Residual spray containing permethrin for application by ground crew.

Product details: Supplied as emulsifiable concentrate formulation (50%), to be diluted to 2% permethrin for use. The application rate is 0.2 grams permethrin/m^2 for internal surfaces (0.5 grams/m^2 for floors).

Evaluation of formulation components: With the exception of permethrin the components of the formulation were not considered to present a particular concern for human health.

Assessment against WHO criteria: The formulation and spray rate comply with WHO recommendations.

Alternative presentations of this product type: This type of product can also be supplied in a ready-to-use form (as a 2% solution). Due to the absence of exposure via mixing and loading operations, exposures of ground crew from the ready-to-use form are expected to be lower than the exposures presented in the following evaluation.

This type of product may also be applied via a semi-automated fogging device while the aircraft is empty. Since personnel will not be present during application with this device, exposures of ground crew are also expected to be lower than those exposures presented in the following evaluation.

Since the following evaluation is considered to be 'worst-case' relative to these alternative formulations and methods for this product type, separate evaluations are not presented.

Generic risk assessment model	Residual spray concentrate product (permethrin)
1. Toxicity data Aim: To assess available toxicity data and derive acceptable exposure levels	**1. Toxicity data** Aim: To assess available toxicity data and derive acceptable exposure levels
1.1 Conduct literature search for human, animal and in vitro toxicity data and any necessary physicochemical data on the insecticide	1.1 Literature search on permethrin (25:75) conducted on WHO IPCS reviews, JMPR, ATSDR & EFSA
1.2 Obtain relevant reviews and key original papers	1.2 Comprehensive reviews available from IPCS (WHO, 2005), JMPR (JMPR, 1999; JMPR 2002) and IARC (IARC, 1991).
1.3 Tabulate types of study, toxic effects observed, NOAELs and LOAELs.	1.3 All key animal studies tabulated.
1.4 Assess whether quality of database is adequate for risk assessment (range of studies, conduct of studies, adequacy of dose–response data, etc.).	1.4 Studies available on all relevant types of toxicity, most via oral route, with some inhalation and dermal studies. Most conducted to acceptable standards with adequate dose–response data.
1.5 If database is adequate, identify critical toxic effect(s).	1.5 In humans, first symptom of exposure is facial paraesthesia, reversible on cessation of exposure. Critical toxic effect in animal tests is neurotoxicity. Other effects in long-term tests include clinical signs, changes in body weight and ovary weight. No dose response data are available for humans but database from animals is adequate.
1.6 If the insecticide is a skin or respiratory sensitizer, is genotoxic, carcinogenic or extremely acutely toxic, consider whether it is worth proceeding with risk assessment. Consider this also if it produces clear	1.6 Permethrin is not genotoxic, and has not shown carcinogenic or specific reproductive toxic effects. Skin sensitization tests have been negative and no cases of skin or respiratory tract sensitization are reported in the scientific literature despite previous use in different applications. Permethrin was slightly irritating to skin and mildly irritating to eyes. Permethrin has moderate acute toxicity. Toxicokinetic data

Generic risk assessment model	Residual spray concentrate product (permethrin)
reproductive toxic effects at dose levels causing no general toxicity.	suggests good oral absorption. Default 100% oral absorption is used in this assessment. Proceed with risk assessment.
1.7 If 1.6 does not apply, identify pivotal study/studies giving dose–response data for critical effect(s).	1.7 Pivotal studies are: – 1-year dog oral study – 2-year rat oral study – acute rat oral neurotoxicity study
1.8 Identify critical NOAEL(s) from pivotal studies for acute exposure and for longer-term (repeat-dose) exposure.	1.8 Critical NOAELs are: – 1-year oral study, dog, NOAEL = 5 mg/kg bw per day – 2-year oral study, rat, NOAEL= 5 mg/kg bw per day – acute rat neurotoxicity study, NOAEL = 150 mg/kg bw
1.9 Assess whether the database allows the setting of TSDs for short-term and long-term exposures.	1.9 Database adequate to allow setting of TSD for single and repeated exposures.
1.10 Set TSDs for oral, dermal or inhalation exposure by dividing NOAEL for the critical effect from the pivotal study via that route by an uncertainty factor (UF): TSD = NOAEL/UF (correcting for systemic bioavailability if necessary). A default UF of 100 is recommended for NOAELs derived from animal studies and 10 for NOAELs derived from human studies.	1.10 The ADI of 0.05 mg/kg bw per day is set by JMPR (JMPR, 1999). This is based on a 1-year oral dog study and a 2 year rat study, in which NOAELs of 5 mg/kg bw per day were identified. Application of a UF of 100 to the lowest NOAEL, 5 mg/kg bw per day, results in a TSD of 0.05 mg/kg bw per day. JMPR has also set an ARfD of 1.5 mg/kg bw (JMPR, 2002). This is based on a rat acute oral neurotoxicity study in which an NOAEL of 150 mg/kg bw was identified.
1.11 Conclusion on final TSD(s).	1.11 TSDs used in risk characterization: – long-term TSD, 0.05 mg/kg bw per day – short-term TSD_{AC}, 1.5 mg/kg bw

Generic risk assessment model	Residual spray concentrate product (permethrin)
2. Exposure assessment *Aim:* – to estimate occupational exposure via dermal and inhalation routes during mixing, loading and application of residual sprays in an aircraft for disinsection purposes; – to estimate exposure of adult and child passengers (post-application inhalation and dermal exposure, and toddlers' hand-to-mouth exposure). 10% default is used for dermal absorption 100% default is used for inhalation and gastrointestinal absorption Protection factor of adequate protective equipment, including gloves, is assumed to be 90%. Body weight is 62 kg for adults, 32 kg for older children and 14 kg for toddlers.	**2. Exposure assessment: residual product** An emulsifiable concentrate formulation of permethrin 25:75 is to be applied to residual spraying. Product only used as a surface spray. The concentration of a.i. in the formulation as supplied is 50%, which is diluted with water to 2% a.i. for the spray solution. The target concentration on surfaces is 0.2 g permethrin/m^2 for interior surfaces and 0.4–0.5 g permethrin/m^2 for floors (essentially the floor is treated twice with the spray solution). The application rate of spray solution is 10 ml/m^2. The guideline scenarios represent a situation where label instructions are being followed. In the lax standard scenarios, it may be assumed, for example, that no gloves are used or that spraying equipment is not totally leakproof.
2.1 Ground crew operator exposure *a) Mixing and loading* In mixing and loading, only dermal exposure is considered significant. It is assumed that the amount of the spray liquid prepared per day to treat the interior	**2.1 Ground crew operator exposure** *a) Mixing and loading* Product used is a 2% emulsion, diluted from 50% a.i. by ground staff or authorised applicators. Chronic systemic dose due to dermal exposure, mg a.i./kg bw per day: 0.04 ml × 500 mg a.i./ml × 1.0 × 10% × 104 days/(62 kg × 365 days)

Generic risk assessment model	Residual spray concentrate product (permethrin)
surfaces of a large aircraft is three 10-litre tanks. The floors are treated twice. For the purposes of the calculations the floor area is assumed to be one-third of the interior surface. This requires an additional 10-litre tank. It is also assumed that ground personnel need to spray an aeroplane twice a week throughout the year. In the guideline scenario, gloves are used. In the lax standard scenario, no gloves are assumed. Default values for hand contamination while mixing and loading are available (0.01 ml/operation).	= **0.009 mg a.i./kg bw per day** (lax standard scenario). In guideline scenario calculation, a protection factor of 90% applies, hence the systemic dose is: 0.04 ml × 500 mg a.i./ml × 0.1 × 10% × 104 days/(62 kg × 365 days) = **0.0009 mg a.i./kg bw per day** The maximum daily systemic dose will be: 0.04 ml × 500 mg a.i./ml × 1.0 × 10%/62 kg = **0.032 mg/kg bw** (lax standard scenario) 0.04 ml × 500 mg a.i./ml × 0.1 × 10%/62 kg = **0.0032 mg/kg bw** (guideline scenario)
b) Application The quantity of spray to be applied depends on the area of the internal surfaces of the aircraft. A large aircraft with an internal surface area of 2500 m^2 and a volume of 1000 m^3 is assumed for these calculations. The required dosage is 0.2 g a.i./m^2 for interior surfaces and 0.4–0.5 g a.i./m^2 for floors. With the 2% preparation, 10 ml of the spray liquid must be applied per square metre. With a sprayer adjusted to deliver 10 ml/s, the correct deposit will be achieved if	*b) Application* As the spray liquid is 2% emulsion, the spray concentration will be 20 mg/ml. Concentration of the aerosol in the inhaled air: 10 ml of spray is applied/m^2, which in a large aircraft means that 25 litres, or 25 000 ml, of spray liquid is needed. Approximately 0.1% of the sprayed a.i. is assumed to be evenly distributed in the air, i.e. in a volume of 1000 m^3. The inhalable concentration (CA) of the aerosol would then be 0.001 × 25 000/1000 ml/m^3 = 0.025 ml of spray/m^3. Systemic dose due to inhalation exposure, mg a.i./kg bw per day: 20 mg/ml × 0.025 ml/m^3 × 1.0 × 3.8 m^3 × 100% × 104 days/(62 kg × 365 days) = **0.0087 mg a.i./kg bw per day** (lax standard scenario) In the guideline scenario, the use of protective equipment provides a 90% protection factor.

Generic risk assessment model	Residual spray concentrate product (permethrin)
one square metre is sprayed per second. The floors are treated twice. It is assumed, that 9.3 ml of spray liquid will contaminate hands during one work day. Breathing rate 1.9 m³/hour, work time 2 hours – air volume inhaled = 3.8 m³. It is assumed that 0.1% of the a.i. sprayed will be evenly distributed in the air (including in the breathing zone of the operator). The default absorption rate from the respiratory tract is 100%.	The exposure will therefore be 10% of that in the lax standard scenario, i.e. **0.00087 mg a.i./kg bw per day** The maximum daily systemic dose will be: 20 mg/ml × 0.025 ml/m³ × 1.0 × 3.8 m³ × 100%/62 = **0.031 mg a.i./kg bw** (lax standard scenario) 20 mg/ml × 0.025 ml/m³ × 0.1 × 3.8 m³ × 100%/62 = **0.0031 mg a.i./kg bw** (guideline scenario) Systemic dose due to dermal exposure, mg a.i./kg bw per day: 9.3 ml/day × 20 mg/ml × 1.0 × 10% × 104 days/(62 kg × 365 days) = **0.085 mg a.i./kg bw per day** (lax standard scenario) In the guideline scenario calculation, the protection factor for protective clothing (90%) is applied, and the systemic dose is **0.0085 mg a.i./kg bw per day** The maximum daily systemic dose will be: 9.3 ml/day × 20 mg/ml × 1.0 × 10%/62 kg = **0.3 mg a.i./kg bw** (lax standard scenario) 9.3 ml/day × 20 mg/ml × 0.1 × 10%/62 kg = **0.03 mg a.i./kg bw** (guideline scenario)
2.2 Cabin crew and passenger exposure from residual disinsection Passenger and cabin crew exposure is assumed to be due to secondary dermal exposure from contact with the surfaces of the aircraft. For passengers and cabin crew, the proportion translodged onto bare skin is 11%; the exposed area of skin reflects the clothing worn, with an additional component for toddlers because of greater activity.	**2.2 Cabin crew and passenger exposure from residual disinsection** Product specific target concentration on the surfaces, 0.2 g/m² = 200 mg/m². The higher dose applied to floors is balanced by lower transfer from carpet to skin (USEPA, 2009), hence all calculations can be based on 0.2 g/m². Systemic dose of cabin crew members due to dermal exposure, mg a.i./kg bw per day: 200 mg/m² × 11% × 0.1 m² × 10% × 240 days/(62 kg × 365 days) = **0.002 mg a.i./kg bw** Maximum daily exposure: 200 mg/m² × 11% × 0.1 m² × 10%/62 kg

Generic risk assessment model	Residual spray concentrate product (permethrin)
For cabin crew, the exposed skin area is 0.1 m^2 (50% of hands and forearms) and the exposure duration is 240 days per year. For passengers, the exposed skin areas are 0.25 m^2 for adults, 0.16 m^2 for older children, and 0.2 m^2 for toddlers. Exposure duration is 40 days for adult passengers and 5 days for children. In addition, the sprayed insecticide may be dislodged from surfaces as contaminated dust leading to ingestion by toddlers due to hand-to-mouth behaviour. For estimating the hand-to-mouth exposure, the relevant hand area for toddlers is 0.032 m^2. For the extent of the transfer from hands to mouth, a default of 10% is used.	= **0.0035 mg a.i./kg bw.** Systemic dose of the passengers due to dermal exposure, mg a.i./kg bw per day: 200 mg/m^2 × 11% × (0.25 m^2, 0.16 m^2 or 0.2 m^2) × 10% × (40 days or 5 days)/((62 kg, 32 kg or 14 kg) × 365 days) Long-term exposures: for adults: **0.00097 mg a.i./kg bw per day** for children: **0.00015 mg a.i./kg bw per day** for toddlers: **0.00043 mg a.i./kg bw per day** Maximum daily exposures: for adults: **0.0088 mg a.i./kg bw** for children: **0.011 mg a.i./kg bw** for toddlers: **0.031 mg a.i./kg bw** Systemic dose due to hand-to-mouth behaviour, toddlers, mg a.i./kg bw per day: 200 mg/m^2 × 11% × 0.032 m^2 × 10% × 100% × 5 days/(14 kg × 365 days) = **0.00007 mg a.i./kg bw per day** Maximum daily exposure: 200 mg/m^2 × 11% × 0.032 m^2 × 10% × 100%/14 kg = **0.005 mg a.i./kg bw**
3. Risk characterization 3.1 Compare exposure estimates with TSDs for risk characterization. For products with appreciable acute toxicity, comparison against TSD_{AC} should also be considered. 3.2 If the exposure calculated for a subgroup and exposure route is below the respective TSD, using conservative estimates, it can be	**3. Risk characterization** Permethrin has moderate acute toxicity. Thus the risk assessment is based on:- – comparison of chronic exposure with the long-term TSD; – comparison of acute exposure with the short-term TSD_{AC}. From section 1.10, the TSD used in long-term risk characterization is 0.05 mg/kg bw per day. Short-term guidance value (TSD_{AC}) is 1.5 mg/kg bw.

Generic risk assessment model	Residual spray concentrate product (permethrin)
assumed that the exposure is acceptable and does not cause unacceptable risk to human health. 3.3 If the exposure is above the TSD and refining the assessment process, e.g. by use of chemical-specific data, fails to bring the exposure below the TSD, measures to reduce the exposure must be implemented. 3.4 In some cases the exposure may be found to be unacceptable, despite measures to reduce it. Other methods of vector control should be considered.	**Predicted doses to be used in subsequent risk characterization:** *Total operator predicted dose, ground personnel performing residual disinsections:* • Long-term (TWA) exposure Lax standard scenario: $dose_{M/L}$ dermal + $dose_{A}$ inhalation + $dose_{A}$ dermal = 0.009 + 0.0087 + 0.085 = **0.1 mg a.i./kg bw per day** Guideline scenario: $dose_{M/L}$ dermal + $dose_{A}$ inhalation + $dose_{A}$ dermal = 0.0009 + 0.00087 + 0.0085 = **0.01 mg a.i./kg bw per day** where: $dose_{M/L}$ refers to exposure from mixing and loading, and $dose_{A}$ refers to exposure from application In the guideline exposure scenario, worker exposure is considered to be acceptable, as the total predicted dose is 20% of the TSD. In the lax standard scenario, the TSD may be exceeded by a factor of 2. It is therefore important to make sure that safe practices are implemented, that adequate PPE is used, and that the equipment is maintained in good working condition. • Acute (maximal daily) exposure Lax standard scenario: $dose_{M/L}$ dermal + $dose_{A}$ inhalation + $dose_{A}$ dermal = 0.032 + 0.031 + 0.3 = **0.36 mg a.i./kg bw** Guideline scenario: $dose_{M/L}$ dermal + $dose_{A}$ inhalation + $dose_{A}$ dermal = 0.0032 + 0.0031 + 0.03 = **0.036 mg a.i./kg bw**

Generic risk assessment model	Residual spray concentrate product (permethrin)
	In the guideline exposure scenario, acute worker exposure is considered to be acceptable, as the maximal daily dose is approximately 2% of the TSD_{AC}. Even in the lax standard scenario, acute worker exposure is considered to be acceptable, as the maximum daily dose is approximately 24% of the TSD_{AC}. *Total cabin crew predicted dose:* Dose from touching contaminated surfaces = **0.002 mg a.i./kg bw per day (TWA) or 0.0035 mg a.i./kg bw (maximal daily exposure)** Cabin crew exposure is considered to be acceptable. The predicted doses are less than 5% of the TSD and less than 1% of the TSD_{AC}. *Total passenger predicted doses:* • Long-term exposure for adult passengers **0.00097 mg a.i./kg bw per day** for children **0.00015 mg a.i./kg bw per day** • Maximum daily exposures: for adult passengers **0.0088 mg a.i./kg bw** for children **0.011 mg a.i./kg bw** Exposure of adult and child passengers from residual treatment is considered to be acceptable – the predicted doses are less than 2% of the TSD and less than 1% of the TSD_{AC}. *Total passenger predicted doses – toddlers:* • Long-term dose from touching contaminated surfaces + dose from hand-to-mouth behaviour = 0.00043 + 0.00007 = **0.0005 mg a.i./kg bw per day** • Maximum daily exposure

Generic risk assessment model	Residual spray concentrate product (permethrin)
	from touching contaminated surfaces + dose from hand-to-mouth behaviour = 0.031 + 0.005 = **0.036 mg a.i./kg bw** Exposure of toddlers from residual treatment is considered to be acceptable – the predicted doses represent 1% and less than 3% of the TSD and TSD_{AC}, respectively.

EVALUATION OF SPACE SPRAY AEROSOL PRODUCTS FOR AIRCRAFT HOLD DISINSECTION

Product type: Aerosol spray can product containing d-phenothrin and permethrin for space spraying within the aircraft hold using a single shot lockdown nozzle.

Product details: Aerosol spray can containing 2% d-phenothrin and 2% permethrin. The spray rate equates to 35 grams of formulation per 100 cubic metres.

Evaluation of formulation components: With the exception of d-phenothrin and permethrin the components of the formulation were not considered to present a particular concern for human health.

Assessment against WHO criteria: The formulation and spray rate comply with WHO recommendations.

Generic risk assessment model	Space spray aerosol products for aircraft hold disinsection
1. Toxicity data Aim: To assess available toxicity data and derive acceptable exposure levels	**1. Toxicity data** Aim: To assess available toxicity data and derive acceptable exposure levels
1.1 Conduct literature search for human, animal and in vitro toxicity data and any necessary physicochemical data on the insecticide	1.1 Literature searches on permethrin and d-phenothrin conducted on WHO IPCS reviews, JMPR, ATSDR & EFSA.
1.2 Obtain relevant reviews and key original papers	1.2 Comprehensive reviews available from IPCS (WHO, 2005), JMPR (JMPR 1988, JMPR 1999; JMPR 2002) and IARC (IARC, 1991).
1.3 Tabulate types of study, toxic effects observed, NOAELs and LOAELs.	1.3 All available relevant animal studies tabulated.

Generic risk assessment model	Space spray aerosol products for aircraft hold disinsection
1.4 Assess whether quality of database is adequate for risk assessment (range of studies, conduct of studies, adequacy of dose–response data, etc.).	1.4 Studies available on all relevant types of toxicity, most via oral route, with some inhalation and dermal studies. Most conducted to acceptable standards with adequate dose–response data. JMPR state that the data presented indicate similar metabolism and toxicity for phenothrin and d-phenothrin, thus indicating that data for phenothrin can be used to support the toxicological database for d-phenothrin.
1.5 If database is adequate, identify critical toxic effect(s).	1.5 In humans, first symptom of exposure is facial paraesthesia, reversible on cessation of exposure. Critical toxic effect for both substances in animal tests is neurotoxicity. For permethrin, other effects in long-term tests include clinical signs, changes in body weight and ovary weight. For d-phenothrin, other effects in long-term tests include changes in liver weight, haematology and histopathological alterations in adrenal glands and liver. No dose response data are available for humans but database from animals is adequate.
1.6 If the insecticide is a skin or respiratory sensitizer, is genotoxic, carcinogenic or extremely acutely toxic, consider whether it is worth proceeding with risk assessment. Consider this also if it produces clear reproductive toxic effects at dose levels causing no general toxicity.	1.6 The substances are not genotoxic, and have not shown carcinogenic or specific reproductive toxic effects. Skin sensitization studies were negative. The substances were slightly irritating to skin and mildly irritating to eyes. Permethrin has moderate acute toxicity while d-phenothrin has low acute toxicity. Toxicokinetic data suggests good oral absorption. Default 100% oral absorption is used in this assessment. Proceed with risk assessment.
1.7 If 1.6 does not apply, identify pivotal study/studies giving dose–response data for critical effect(s)	1.7 Pivotal studies are: Permethrin:- – 1-year dog oral study – 2-year rat oral study – acute rat oral neurotoxicity study d-Phenothrin:- – 6-month and 1-year dog oral studies

Generic risk assessment model	Space spray aerosol products for aircraft hold disinsection
1.8 Identify critical NOAEL(s) from pivotal studies for acute exposure and for longer-term (repeat-dose) exposure.	1.8 Critical NOAELs are: Permethrin:- – 1-year oral study, dog, NOAEL = 5 mg/kg bw per day – 2-year oral study, rat, NOAEL= 5 mg/kg bw per day – acute rat neurotoxicity study, NOAEL = 150 mg/kg bw d-Phenothrin:- – 6-month and 1-year oral studies, dog, NOAEL = 7.1 mg/kg bw per day
1.9 Assess whether the database allows the setting of TSDs for short-term and long-term exposures.	1.9 Database adequate to allow setting of TSDs for single (permethrin) and repeated exposures (permethrin and d-phenothrin).
1.10 Set TSDs for oral, dermal or inhalation exposure by dividing NOAEL for the critical effect from the pivotal study via that route by an uncertainty factor (UF): TSD = NOAEL/UF (correcting for systemic bioavailability if necessary). A default UF of 100 is recommended for NOAELs derived from animal studies and 10 for NOAELs derived from human studies.	1.10 Permethrin: The ADI of 0.05 mg/kg bw per day is set by JMPR (JMPR, 1999). This is based on a 1-year oral dog study and a 2 year rat study, in which NOAELs of 5 mg/kg bw per day were identified. Application of a UF of 100 to the lowest NOAEL, 5 mg/kg bw per day, results in a TSD of 0.05 mg/kg bw per day. JMPR has also set an ARfD of 1.5 mg/kg bw (JMPR, 2002). This is based on a rat acute oral neurotoxicity study in which an NOAEL of 150 mg/kg bw was identified. d-Phenothrin: The ADI of 0.07 mg/kg bw per day is set by JMPR (JMPR, 1988). This is based on 6-month and 1-year dog studies, from which an overall NOAEL of 7.1 mg/kg bw per day was derived. Application of UF of 100 to the NOAEL, 7.1 mg/kg bw per day, results in a TSD of 0.07 mg/kg bw per day. No acute reference dose (ARfD) has been set for d-phenothrin (comparison is made against the TSD_{AC} for permethrin).

Generic risk assessment model	Space spray aerosol products for aircraft hold disinsection
1.11 Conclusion on final TSD(s).	1.11 TSDs used in risk characterization: Permethrin:- – long-term TSD, 0.05 mg/kg bw per day – short-term TSD_{AC}, 1.5 mg/kg bw d-Phenothrin:- – long-term TSD, 0.07 mg/kg bw per day
2. Exposure assessment *Aim:* – to estimate occupational exposure via dermal and inhalation routes during application of aerosol sprays in an aircraft hold for disinsection purposes. 10% default is used for dermal absorption. 100% default is used for absorption via the respiratory tract. Protection factor of adequate protective equipment, including gloves, is assumed to be 90% Body weight is 62 kg for adults.	**2. Exposure assessment: aerosol spray product** An aerosol product containing 2% permethrin (25:75) and 2% d-phenothrin (20:80) for space spraying, packed in an aerosol can with a propellant. Spray rate (discharge rate from can) is 2 g/s. The entire contents of the can are discharged when the single shot lockdown nozzle is activated. The guideline scenario represents a situation where label instructions are being followed precisely. In the lax standard scenario, it may be assumed, for example, that no gloves are used or label instructions are not completely complied with.
2.1 Ground crew operator exposure The product is a pre-prepared aerosol spray can containing 2% of each a.i. No mixing and loading is required.	**2.1 Ground crew operator exposure** The product specific parameters required by the inhalation model are: – the mass generation rate, or the amount of compound released from the can during spraying per unit of time (4 g/s to reflect the number of cans being discharged simultaneously in this example scenario);

Generic risk assessment model	Space spray aerosol products for aircraft hold disinsection
For the purposes of this risk assessment a large aircraft (volume 1000 m^3) is assumed, with a scenario of four 150 g cans being discharged (2 cans in each section of the hold). The 'worst-case' scenario of ground crew being required to re-enter the hold after disinsection has taken place (not a routine occurrence) is addressed. This could result in inhalation exposure (30 minutes is assumed) and hand contact with spray residue on surfaces (internal surfaces of the hold or hold contents). Default values for the general exposure parameters needed for inhalation exposure assessment with ConsExpo software are: – the spray duration (in this case estimated 200 seconds); – exposure duration (30 minutes assumed); – room volume (or in this case, volume of large aircraft, default 1000 m^3); – room height (estimated 2 m); – ventilation rate (as a worst case it is assumed that there is no effect due to ventilation).	– estimate of the airborne, non-volatile fraction (a worst-case assumption has been made, that this fraction is 100%); – inhalation cut-off droplet diameter (15 μm); – weight fraction of non-volatiles (default 2%); – weight fraction of compound of interest in the product (percentage of a.i. in the product, 2%); – density of non-volatile compounds (assumed 1.8 g/cm^3); – initial particle distribution (assumed log-normal, average particle diameter 8 μm, coefficient of variation 0.45). Respiration rate of ground crew operators is assumed to be 1.9 m^3/h. Space spray is not intended to settle on surfaces, but is likely to be carried away by the air circulation. It can be assumed that 1% of the material sprayed into the air could be deposited on the surfaces. If four 150 g cans are discharged (600 g spray), containing 2% a.i. (12 g), into a large aircraft with surface area of 2500 m^2, then the amount which settles would be (12 g × 1%)/2500 m^2 = 0.048 mg/m^2. Contact is with 50% of hands and forearms only (0.1 m^2). *Systemic dose due to inhalation exposure:* These exposure estimates are obtained directly from the output of the ConsExpo software. **0.025 mg a.i./kg bw per day** (ConsExpo Output – inhalation chronic systemic dose, point-estimate) **0.038 mg a.i./kg bw per day** (ConsExpo Output – inhalation acute systemic dose, point-estimate) *Systemic dose due to dermal exposure via hands and arms in contact with surfaces:* 0.048 mg/m^2 × 11% × 0.1 m^2 × 240 days × 10%/62 kg × 365 days = **0.000 000 6 mg a.i./kg bw per day**

Generic risk assessment model	Space spray aerosol products for aircraft hold disinsection
	Systemic dose due to dermal exposure via contamination of fingers with spray liquid (leaking nozzle): 1 ml/day × 20 mg/ml × 240 days × 10%/62 kg × 365 days = **0.02 mg a.i./kg bw per day** • Maximum daily exposures from hands and arms in contact with surfaces: 0.048 mg/m^2 × 11% × 0.1 m^2 × 10%/62 kg = **0.000 000 9 mg a.i./kg bw** • Maximum daily exposures from contamination of fingers: 1 ml/day × 20 mg/ml × 10%/62 kg = **0.032 mg a.i./kg bw**
2.2 Space spraying, passenger exposure This type of product is only applied to the aircraft hold.	**2.2 Space spraying, passenger exposure** Not applicable.
3 Risk characterization 3.1 Compare exposure estimates with TSDs for risk characterization. For products with appreciable acute toxicity, consideration should be given to comparing against TSD_{AC}. 3.2 If the exposure calculated for a subgroup and exposure route is below the respective TSD, using conservative estimates, it can be assumed that the exposure is acceptable and does not cause unacceptable risk to human health.	**3 Risk characterization** Permethrin has moderate acute toxicity, d-phenothrin has low acute toxicity. The risk assessment is based on:- – comparison of chronic exposure with the long-term TSD; – comparison of acute exposure with the short-term TSD_{AC}. From section 1.10, the TSD used in long-term risk characterization is 0.05 mg/kg bw per day for permethrin and 0.07 mg/kg bw per day for d-phenothrin. Short-term guidance value (TSA_{AC}) is 1.5 mg/kg bw per day for permethrin; no short-term guidance value has been set for d-phenothrin. **Predicted doses to be used in subsequent risk characterization:** *Total operator predicted dose, ground personnel performing space spraying in the aircraft hold:* • Long-term (TWA) exposure

Generic risk assessment model	Space spray aerosol products for aircraft hold disinsection
3.3 If the exposure is above the TSD and refining the assessment process, e.g. by use of chemical-specific data, fails to bring the exposure below the TSD, measures to reduce the exposure must be implemented 3.4 In some cases the exposure may be found to be unacceptable despite measures to reduce it. Other methods of vector control should be considered.	Guideline scenario: $Inhalation_{dose}$ + Dermal contact with $surfaces_{dose}$ = 0.025 + 0.000 000 6 = **0.025 mg a.i./kg bw per day** Lax standard scenario: $Inhalation_{dose}$ + Dermal contact with $surfaces_{dose}$ + Contamination of $fingers_{dose}$ = 0.025 + 0.000 000 6 + 0.02 = **0.045 mg a.i./kg bw per day** In the guideline scenario, the exposure is approximately 35–50% of the TSDs for permethrin and d-phenothrin. In the lax standard scenario, taking into account contamination of the fingers due to leaking nozzles, the exposure is approximately 64–90% of the TSDs. • Acute (maximal daily) exposure Guideline scenario: $Inhalation_{dose}$ + Dermal contact with $surfaces_{dose}$ = 0.038 + 0.000 000 9 = **0.038 mg a.i./kg bw** Lax standard scenario: $Inhalation_{dose}$ + Dermal contact with $surfaces_{dose}$ + Contamination of $fingers_{dose}$ = 0.038 + 0.000 000 9 + 0.032 = **0.07 mg a.i./kg bw** In both the guideline and lax standard scenarios the exposure is less than 5% of the TSD_{AC} for permethrin. This is considered adequate to cover the acute risk from exposure to d-phenothrin. This risk assessment uses a number of very conservative assumptions. Entry of ground crew into an aircraft hold shortly after disinsection will not be a routine occurrence, hence the assumption of 240 days per year for occupational exposure (and 30 minutes subsequent exposure time) is very conservative. Also, contamination of fingers due to leaking spray nozzles should be very rare in practice.

Generic risk assessment model	Space spray aerosol products for aircraft hold disinsection
	Even with these very conservative assumptions, the predicted exposures for ground crew are all lower than the TSD or TSD_{AC} values and the exposures are considered to be acceptable.

EVALUATION OF SPACE SPRAY AEROSOL PRODUCTS FOR CABIN DISINSECTION (D-PHENOTHRIN)

Product type: Aerosol spray can product containing d-phenothrin for space spraying by cabin crew.

Product details: Aerosol spray can containing 2% d-phenothrin. The spray rate equates to 35 grams of formulation per 100 cubic metres.

Evaluation of formulation components: With the exception of d-phenothrin the components of the formulation were not considered to present a particular concern for human health.

Assessment against WHO criteria: The formulation and spray rate comply with WHO recommendations.

Generic risk assessment model	Space spray aerosol products for cabin disinsection (d-phenothrin)
1. Toxicity data Aim: To assess available toxicity data and derive acceptable exposure levels	**1. Toxicity data** Aim: To assess available toxicity data and derive acceptable exposure levels
1.1 Conduct literature search for human, animal and in vitro toxicity data and any necessary physicochemical data on the insecticide	1.1 Literature search on d-phenothrin conducted on WHO IPCS reviews, JMPR, ATSDR & EFSA.
1.2 Obtain relevant reviews and key original papers	1.2 Comprehensive reviews available from IPCS (WHO, 2005) and JMPR (JMPR, 1988).
1.3 Tabulate types of study, toxic effects observed, NOAELs and LOAELs.	1.3 All available relevant animal studies tabulated.
1.4 Assess whether quality of database is adequate for risk assessment (range of studies, conduct of studies, adequacy of dose–response data, etc.).	1.4 Studies available on all relevant types of toxicity, most via oral route, with some inhalation and dermal studies. Most conducted to acceptable standards with adequate dose–response data. JMPR state that the data presented indicate similar metabolism and

Generic risk assessment model	Space spray aerosol products for cabin disinsection (d-phenothrin)
	toxicity for phenothrin and d-phenothrin, thus indicating that data for phenothrin can be used to support the toxicological database for d-phenothrin.
1.5 If database is adequate, identify critical toxic effect(s).	1.5 In humans, first symptom of exposure is facial paraesthesia, reversible on cessation of exposure. Critical toxic effect in animal tests is neurotoxicity. Other effects in long-term tests include changes in liver weight, haematology and histopathological alterations in adrenal glands and liver. No dose response data are available for humans but database from animals is adequate.
1.6 If the insecticide is a skin or respiratory sensitizer, is genotoxic, carcinogenic or extremely acutely toxic, consider whether it is worth proceeding with risk assessment. Consider this also if it produces clear reproductive toxic effects at dose levels causing no general toxicity.	1.6 d-Phenothrin is not genotoxic, and has not shown carcinogenic or specific reproductive toxic effects. Skin sensitization tests have been negative and no cases of skin or respiratory tract sensitization are reported in the scientific literature despite previous use of the insecticide in different applications. d-Phenothrin has low acute toxicity. Toxicokinetic data suggests good oral absorption. Default 100% oral absorption is used in this assessment. Proceed with risk assessment.
1.7 If 1.6 does not apply, identify pivotal study/studies giving dose–response data for critical effect(s).	1.7 Pivotal studies are: – 6-month and 1-year dog oral studies
1.8 Identify critical NOAEL(s) from pivotal studies for acute exposure and for longer-term (repeat-dose) exposure.	1.8 Critical NOAELs are: – 6-month and 1-year oral studies, dog, NOAEL = 7.1 mg/kg bw per day
1.9 Assess whether the database allows the setting of TSDs for short-term and long-term exposures.	1.9 Database adequate to allow setting of TSD.
1.10 Set TSDs for oral, dermal or inhalation	1.10 The ADI of 0.07 mg/kg bw per day is set by JMPR (JMPR, 1988). This is based on

Generic risk assessment model	Space spray aerosol products for cabin disinsection (d-phenothrin)
exposure by dividing NOAEL for the critical effect from the pivotal study via that route by an uncertainty factor (UF): TSD = NOAEL/UF (correcting for systemic bioavailability if necessary). A default UF of 100 is recommended for NOAELs derived from animal studies and 10 for NOAELs derived from human studies.	6-month and 1-year dog studies, from which an overall NOAEL of 7.1 mg/kg bw per day was derived. Application of UF of 100 to the NOAEL, 7.1 mg/kg bw per day, results in a TSD of 0.07 mg/kg bw per day. No acute reference dose (ARfD) has been set for d-phenothrin (comparison can be made against the TSD_{AC} for another pyrethroid insecticide – permethrin).
1.11 Conclusion on final TSD(s).	1.11 TSDs used in risk characterization: – long-term TSD, 0.07 mg/kg bw per day – short-term TSD_{AC}, 1.5 mg/kg bw (from permethrin)
2. Exposure assessment *Aim:* – to estimate occupational exposure via dermal and inhalation routes resulting from spraying aerosol sprays in an aircraft for disinsection purposes; – to estimate exposure of adult and child passengers (post-application inhalation and dermal exposure, and toddlers' hand-to-mouth exposure). 10% default is used for dermal absorption 100% default is used for inhalation and gastrointestinal absorption	**2. Exposure assessment: aerosol spray product** An aerosol product containing 2% d-phenothrin (20:80) for space spraying, packed in an aerosol can with a propellant. Spray rate (discharge rate from can) is 0.8–1.2 g/s. For the purposes of this risk assessment a large aircraft (volume 1000 m^3) is assumed, with a scenario of four 100 g cans being discharged. The guideline scenarios represent a situation where label instructions are being followed and assume that the products used are in good working order Touching surfaces is the only source of dermal exposure in the guideline scenario. In the lax standard scenario the spray nozzle may leak leading to fingers becoming contaminated.

Generic risk assessment model	Space spray aerosol products for cabin disinsection (d-phenothrin)
Body weight is 62 kg for adults, 32 kg for older children and 14 kg for toddlers.	
2.1 Space spraying, cabin crew exposure, application Default values for the general exposure parameters needed for inhalation exposure assessment with ConsExpo software are: – the spray duration (in this case estimated 200 seconds); – exposure duration (30 minutes); – room volume (or in this case, volume of the cabin, large aircraft, default 1000 m^3); – room height (estimated 2 m); – ventilation rate (as a worst case it is assumed that there is no effect due to ventilation). The remaining parameters needed for the software are product-specific. Respiration rate of cabin crew members is assumed to be 0.89 m^3/h. Space spray is not intended to settle on	***2.1 Space spraying, cabin crew exposure, application*** The product specific parameters required by the ConsExpo inhalation model are: – the mass generation rate, or the amount of compound released from the can during spraying per unit of time (2 g/s to reflect two cans being discharged simultaneously in this example scenario); – estimate of the airborne, non-volatile fraction (a worst-case assumption has been made, that this fraction is 100%); – inhalation cut-off droplet diameter (15 μm); – weight fraction of non-volatiles (default 2%); – weight fraction of compound of interest in the product (percentage of a.i. in the product, 2%); – density of non-volatile compounds (assumed 1.8 g/cm^3); – initial particle distribution (assumed log-normal, average particle diameter 8 μm, coefficient of variation 0.45). *Systemic dose due to inhalation exposure:* These exposure estimates are obtained directly from the output of the ConsExpo software. **0.012 mg a.i./kg bw per day** (ConsExpo Output – inhalation chronic systemic dose, point-estimate) **0.019 mg a.i./kg bw per day** (ConsExpo Output – inhalation acute systemic dose, point-estimate) *Systemic dose due to dermal exposure via body areas in contact with surfaces:*

Generic risk assessment model	Space spray aerosol products for cabin disinsection (d-phenothrin)
surfaces, but is likely to be carried away by the air circulation. It can be assumed that 1% of the material sprayed into the air could be deposited on the surfaces. If four 100 g cans are discharged (400 g spray), containing 2% a.i. (8 g), into a large aircraft with a surface area of 2500 m^2, then the amount which settles would be (8 g × 1%)/2500 m^2 = 0.032 mg/m^2.	0.032 mg/m^2 × 11% × 0.1 m^2 × 240 days × 10%/62 kg × 365 days = **0.000 000 4 mg a.i./kg bw per day** *Systemic dose due to dermal exposure via contamination of fingers with spray liquid (leaking nozzle):* 1 ml/day × 20 mg/ml × 240 days × 10%/62 kg × 365 days =**0.02 mg a.i./kg bw per day** For guideline scenario, systemic dose due to dermal exposure = contact with surfaces only = **0.000 000 4 mg a.i./kg bw per day** For lax standard scenario, systemic dose due to dermal exposure = contact with surfaces + contamination of fingers = 0.000 000 4 + 0.02 = **0.02 mg a.i./kg bw per day** • Maximum daily exposures from body areas in contact with surfaces: 0.032 mg/m^2 × 11% × 0.1 m^2 × 10%/62 kg = **0.000 000 6 mg a.i./kg bw** • Maximum daily exposures from contamination of fingers: 1 ml/day × 20 mg/ml × 10%/62 kg = **0.032 mg a.i./kg bw** For guideline scenario, maximum daily exposure is: **0.000 000 6 mg a.i./kg bw** For lax standard scenario, maximum daily exposure is: 0.000 000 6 + 0.032 = **0.032 mg a.i./kg bw**
2.2 Space spraying, passenger exposure For the systemic dose due to indirect dermal exposure (to material deposited on surfaces), exposed skin areas are 0.25 m^{2}for	***2.2 Space spraying, passenger exposure*** *Systemic dose due to indirect dermal exposure (passengers not present during space spraying – body areas in contact with surfaces where material has deposited):*

Generic risk assessment model	Space spray aerosol products for cabin disinsection (d-phenothrin)
adults, 0.16 m² for older children, 0.2 m² for toddlers. The material deposited on surfaces is calculated in the same way as for cabin crew. If passengers are present during space spraying, the pattern of inhalation exposure is considered to be similar to crew members' exposure. Exposure frequencies are 40 days/year for adult passengers and 5 days/year for children of all ages. See model parameters used in cabin crew exposure calculations. Breathing rates (resting rates) for adult passengers are 0.40 m³/h, for children 6–11 years and toddlers 0.38 m³/h, and for newborn infants 0.28 m³/h. For the systemic dose due to direct dermal contact with the spray, exposed skin areas are 0.33 m² for adults, 0.26 m² for older children, and 0.15 m² for toddlers (based on the head and half of the hands, forearms and lower legs). For newborn infants, only inhalation exposure is considered to be relevant because infants will be held or transported in their own carriers and will have very	0.032 mg/m² × 11% × (0.25, 0.16 or 0.2 m²) × (40 or 5 days) × 10%/(62, 32 or 14 kg) × 365 days (chronic exposure) for adult passengers **0.000 000 2 mg a.i./kg bw per day** for children **0.000 000 03 mg a.i./kg bw per day** for toddlers **0.000 000 07 mg a.i./kg bw per day** • Maximal daily exposure 0.032 mg/m² × 11% × (0.25, 0.16 or 0.2 m²) × 10%/(62, 32 or 14 kg) for adult passengers **0.000 001 4 mg a.i./kg bw** for children **0.000 001 8 mg a.i./kg bw** for toddlers **0.000 005 mg a.i./kg bw** *Systemic dose due to inhalation exposure (passengers present during space spraying):* The exposure estimates are obtained directly from the output of the ConsExpo software. The underlying algorithms are not shown in this worked example: for adult passengers **0.000 93 mg a.i./kg bw per day (chronic)** **0.0085 mg a.i./kg bw (acute)** for children **0.000 21 mg a.i./kg bw per day (chronic)** **0.016 mg a.i./kg bw (acute)** for toddlers **0.000 51 mg a.i./kg bw per day (chronic)** **0.038 mg a.i./kg bw (acute)** for newborn infants **0.0011 mg a.i./kg bw per day (chronic)** **0.077 mg a.i./kg bw (acute)** (ConsExpo Output – inhalation systemic doses, point-estimates) *Systemic dose due to direct skin contact with the spray (passengers present during space spraying:*

Generic risk assessment model	Space spray aerosol products for cabin disinsection (d-phenothrin)
limited opportunity for contact with aircraft surfaces.	0.032 mg/m^2 × (0.33, 0.26 or 0.15 m^2 × (40 or 5 days) × 10%/(62, 32 or 14 kg) × 365 days (chronic exposure) for adult passengers **0.000 002 mg a.i./kg bw per day** for children **0.000 000 4 mg a.i./kg bw per day** for toddlers **0.000 000 5 mg a.i./kg bw per day** • Maximal daily exposure 0.032 mg/m^2 × (0.33, 0.26 or 0.15 m^2 × 10%/(62, 32 or 14 kg) for adult passengers **0.000 017 mg a.i./kg bw** for children **0.000 026 mg a.i./kg bw** for toddlers **0.000 034 mg a.i./kg bw**
3. Risk characterization	**3. Risk characterization**
3.1 Compare exposure estimates with TSDs for risk characterization. For products with appreciable acute toxicity, consideration should be given to comparing against TSD_{AC}. 3.2 If the exposure calculated for a subgroup and exposure route is below the respective TSD, using conservative estimates, it can be assumed that the exposure is acceptable and does not cause unacceptable risk to human health. 3.3 If the exposure is above the TSD and refining the	The risk assessment is based on:- – comparison of chronic exposure with the long-term TSD; – comparison of acute exposure with the short-term TSD_{AC} From section 1.10, the TSD used in long-term risk characterization is 0.07 mg/kg bw per day for d-phenothrin. A short-term guidance value (TSD_{AC}) is not available for d-phenothrin; comparison is made against the TSD_{AC} for permethrin of 1.5 mg/kg bw. ***Predicted doses to be used in subsequent risk characterization*** *Total predicted dose, cabin crew performing space spraying* • Long-term (TWA) exposure

Generic risk assessment model	Space spray aerosol products for cabin disinsection (d-phenothrin)
assessment process, e.g. by use of chemical-specific data, fails to bring the exposure below the TSD, measures to reduce the exposure must be implemented 3.4 In some cases the exposure may be found to be unacceptable despite measures to reduce it. Other methods of vector control should be considered.	Lax standard scenario: $Inhalation_{dose}$ + Dermal contact with $surfaces_{dose}$ + Contamination of $fingers_{dose}$ = 0.012 + 0.000 000 4 + 0.02 = **0.032 mg a.i./kg bw per day** Guideline scenario: $Inhalation_{dose}$ + Dermal contact with $surfaces_{dose}$ = 0.012 + 0.000 000 4 = **0.012 mg a.i./kg bw/day** In the guideline exposure scenario, the exposure is 17% of the TSD. In the lax standard scenario, the predicted exposure is 46% of the TSD. • Acute (maximal daily) exposure Lax standard scenario: $Inhalation_{dose}$ + Dermal contact with $surfaces_{dose}$ + Contamination of $fingers_{dose}$ = 0.019 + 0.000 000 6 + 0.032 = **0.051 mg a.i./kg bw** Guideline scenario: $Inhalation_{dose}$ + Dermal contact with $surfaces_{dose}$ = 0.019 + 0.000 000 6 = **0.019 mg a.i./kg bw** Whilst there is no TSD_{AC} for d-phenothrin the predicted acute exposure is less than 5% of the TSD_{AC} for permethrin in all scenarios. *Predicted doses for passengers from indirect exposure* In this scenario passengers were not present when spraying was carried out and they are exposed through touching surfaces contaminated with spray deposit: for adult passengers **0.000 000 2 mg a.i./kg bw per day (chronic)** **0.000 001 4 mg a.i./kg bw (acute)** for children **0.000 000 02 mg a.i./kg bw per day (chronic)** **0.000 001 8 mg a.i./kg bw (acute)** for toddlers **0.000 000 07 mg a.i./kg bw per day (chronic)** **0.000 005 mg a.i./kg bw (acute)**

Generic risk assessment model	Space spray aerosol products for cabin disinsection (d-phenothrin)
	In all cases these exposures are considered to be acceptable on a chronic basis because the predicted doses are well below the TSD (less than 1%). Whilst there is no TSD_{AC} for d-phenothrin the predicted acute exposure is less than 1% of the TSD_{AC} for permethrin in all cases. *Predicted doses for passengers from direct exposure* In this scenario passengers are present when spraying is carried out and they are exposed through inhalation and also through direct skin contact with the spray while spraying is taking place: for adult passengers $Inhalation_{dose}$ + Skin contact with $spray_{dose}$ = 0.000 93 + 0.000 002 = **0.000 93 mg a.i./kg bw per day (chronic)** This is less than 2% of the TSD. $Inhalation_{dose}$ + Skin contact with $spray_{dose}$ = 0.008 5 + 0.000 017 = **0.008 5 mg a.i./kg bw (acute)** for children $Inhalation_{dose}$ + Skin contact with $spray_{dose}$ = 0.000 21 + 0.000 000 4 = **0.000 21 mg a.i./kg bw per day (chronic)** This is less than 1% of the TSD. $Inhalation_{dose}$ + Skin contact with $spray_{dose}$ = 0.016 + 0.000 026 = **0.016 mg a.i./kg bw (acute)** for toddlers $Inhalation_{dose}$ + Skin contact with $spray_{dose}$ = 0.000 51 + 0.000 000 5 = **0.000 51 mg a.i./kg bw per day (chronic)** This is less than 1% of the TSD. $Inhalation_{dose}$ + Skin contact with $spray_{dose}$ = 0.038 + 0.000 034 = **0.038 mg a.i./kg bw (acute)** For infants $Inhalation_{dose}$ = **0.0011 mg a.i./kg bw per day (chronic)** = **0.077 mg a.i./kg bw (acute)**

Generic risk assessment model	Space spray aerosol products for cabin disinsection (d-phenothrin)
	Exposure of newborn infants is less than 2% of the TSD on a chronic basis. *Assessment* Occupational exposures (cabin crew) on a chronic basis are below the TSD for the guideline and lax standard scenarios. For acute exposures a TSD_{AC} for d-phenothrin is not available but all exposures are less than 5% of the TSD_{AC} for permethrin which is considered to be adequate for this assessment. For passengers, exposures from indirect or direct exposure to spray on a chronic basis are less than 2% of the TSD in all cases. Acute exposures are all less than 5% of the TSD_{AC} for permethrin which is considered to be adequate for this assessment.

EVALUATION OF SPACE SPRAY AEROSOL PRODUCTS FOR CABIN DISINSECTION (PERMETHRIN)

Product type: Aerosol spray can product containing permethrin for space spraying by cabin crew.

Product details: Aerosol spray can containing 2% permethrin. The spray rate equates to 35 grams of formulation per 100 cubic metres.

Evaluation of formulation components: With the exception of permethrin the components of the formulation were not considered to present a particular concern for human health.

Assessment against WHO criteria: The formulation and spray rate comply with WHO recommendations.

Generic risk assessment model	Space spray aerosol products for cabin disinsection (permethrin)
1. Toxicity data	**1. Toxicity data**
Aim: To assess available toxicity data and derive acceptable exposure levels	Aim: To assess available toxicity data and derive acceptable exposure levels
1.1 Conduct literature search for human, animal and in vitro toxicity data and any necessary physicochemical data on the insecticide	1.1 Literature search on permethrin (25:75) conducted on WHO IPCS reviews, JMPR, ATSDR & EFSA
1.2 Obtain relevant reviews and key original papers	1.2 Comprehensive reviews available from IPCS (WHO, 2005), JMPR (JMPR, 1999; JMPR, 2002) and IARC (IARC, 1991).
1.3 Tabulate types of study, toxic effects observed, NOAELs and LOAELs.	1.3 All key animal studies tabulated.
1.4 Assess whether quality of database is adequate for risk assessment (range of studies, conduct of studies, adequacy of dose–response data, etc.).	1.4 Studies available on all relevant types of toxicity, most via oral route, with some inhalation and dermal studies. Most conducted to acceptable standards with adequate dose–response data.

Generic risk assessment model	Space spray aerosol products for cabin disinsection (permethrin)
1.5 If database is adequate, identify critical toxic effect(s).	1.5 In humans, first symptom of exposure is facial paraesthesia, reversible on cessation of exposure. Critical toxic effect in animal tests is neurotoxicity. Other effects in long-term tests include clinical signs, changes in body weight and ovary weight. No dose response data are available for humans but database from animals is adequate.
1.6 If the insecticide is a skin or respiratory sensitizer, is genotoxic, carcinogenic or extremely acutely toxic, consider whether it is worth proceeding with risk assessment. Consider this also if it produces clear reproductive toxic effects at dose levels causing no general toxicity.	1.6 Permethrin is not genotoxic, and has not shown carcinogenic or specific reproductive toxic effects. Skin sensitization tests have been negative and no cases of skin or respiratory tract sensitization are reported in the scientific literature despite previous use in different applications. Permethrin was slightly irritating to skin and mildly irritating to eyes. Permethrin has moderate acute toxicity. Toxicokinetic data suggests good oral absorption. Default 100% oral absorption is used in this assessment. Proceed with risk assessment.
1.7 If 1.6 does not apply, identify pivotal study/studies giving dose–response data for critical effect(s).	1.7 Pivotal studies are: – 1-year dog oral study – 2-year rat oral study – acute rat oral neurotoxicity study
1.8 Identify critical NOAEL(s) from pivotal studies for acute exposure and for longer-term (repeat-dose) exposure.	1.8 Critical NOAELs are: – 1-year oral study, dog, NOAEL = 5 mg/kg bw per day. – 2-year oral study, rat, NOAEL= 5 mg/kg bw per day. – acute rat neurotoxicity study, NOAEL = 150 mg/kg bw
1.9 Assess whether the database allows the setting of TSDs for short-term and long-term exposures.	1.9 Database adequate to allow setting of TSD for single and repeated exposures.
1.10 Set TSDs for oral, dermal or inhalation exposure by dividing NOAEL for the critical	1.10 The ADI of 0.05 mg/kg bw per day is set by JMPR (JMPR, 1999). This is based on a 1-year oral dog study and a 2 year rat study, in which NOAELs of 5 mg/kg bw per day were

Generic risk assessment model	Space spray aerosol products for cabin disinsection (permethrin)
effect from the pivotal study via that route by an uncertainty factor (UF): TSD = NOAEL/UF (correcting for systemic bioavailability if necessary). A default UF of 100 is recommended for NOAELs derived from animal studies and 10 for NOAELs derived from human studies.	identified. Application of a UF of 100 to the lowest NOAEL, 5 mg/kg bw per day, results in a TSD of 0.05 mg/kg bw per day. JMPR has also set an ARfD of 1.5 mg/kg bw (JMPR, 2002). This is based on a rat acute oral neurotoxicity study in which an NOAEL of 150 mg/kg bw was identified.
1.11 Conclusion on final TSD(s).	1.11 TSDs used in risk characterization: – long-term TSD, 0.05 mg/kg bw per day – short-term TSD_{AC}, 1.5 mg/kg bw
2. Exposure assessment *Aim:* – to estimate occupational exposure via dermal and inhalation routes resulting from spraying aerosol sprays in an aircraft for disinsection purposes; – to estimate exposure of adult and child passengers (post-application inhalation and dermal exposure, and toddlers' hand-to-mouth exposure). 10% default is used for dermal absorption 100% default is used for inhalation and gastrointestinal absorption Body weight is 62 kg for adults, 32 kg for older children and 14 kg for toddlers.	**2. Exposure assessment: aerosol spray product** An aerosol product containing 2% permethrin for space spraying, packed in an aerosol can with a propellant. Spray rate (discharge rate from can) is 1 g/s. For the purposes of this risk assessment a large aircraft (volume 1000 m^3) is assumed, with a scenario of four 100 g cans being discharged. The guideline scenarios represent a situation where label instructions are being followed and assume that the products used are in good working order Touching surfaces is the only source of dermal exposure in the guideline scenario. In the lax standard scenario the spray nozzle may leak leading to fingers becoming contaminated.

Generic risk assessment model	Space spray aerosol products for cabin disinsection (permethrin)
2.1 Space spraying, cabin crew exposure, application The exposure model and the parameters are identical to those presented for "*Space spray aerosol products for cabin disinsection (d-phenothrin)*" in an earlier section in this publication.	***2.1 Space spraying, cabin crew exposure, application*** The exposure model and the parameters are identical to those presented for "*Space spray aerosol products for cabin disinsection (d-phenothrin)*" in an earlier section in this publication.
2.2 Space spraying, passenger exposure The exposure model and the parameters are identical to those presented for "*Space spray aerosol products for cabin disinsection (d-phenothrin)*" in an earlier section in this publication.	***2.2 Space spraying, passenger exposure*** The exposure model and the parameters are identical to those presented for "*Space spray aerosol products for cabin disinsection (d-phenothrin)*" in an earlier section in this publication.
3. Risk characterization 3.1 Compare exposure estimates with TSDs for risk characterization. For products with appreciable acute toxicity, consideration should be given to comparing against TSD_{AC}. 3.2 If the exposure calculated for a subgroup and exposure route is below the respective TSD, using conservative estimates, it can be assumed that the exposure is acceptable and does not cause unacceptable risk to human health. 3.3 If the exposure is above the TSD and refining the assessment process, e.g. by use of chemical-specific data, fails to bring	***3. Risk characterization*** The risk assessment is based on:- – comparison of chronic exposure with the long-term TSD; – comparison of acute exposure with the short-term TSD_{AC}. From section 1.10, the TSD used in long-term risk characterization is 0.05 mg/kg bw per day for permethrin. Short-term guidance value (TSD_{AC}) is 1.5 mg/kg bw. ***Predicted doses to be used in subsequent risk characterization:*** *Total predicted dose, cabin crew performing space spraying:* • Long-term (TWA) exposure Lax standard scenario: $Inhalation_{dose}$ + Dermal contact with $surfaces_{dose}$ + Contamination of $fingers_{dose}$ = 0.012 + 0.000 000 4 + 0.02 = **0.032 mg a.i./kg bw per day**

Generic risk assessment model	Space spray aerosol products for cabin disinsection (permethrin)
the exposure below the TSD, measures to reduce the exposure must be implemented 3.4 In some cases the exposure may be found to be unacceptable despite measures to reduce it. Other methods of vector control should be considered.	Guideline scenario: $Inhalation_{dose}$ + Dermal contact with $surfaces_{dose}$ = 0.012 + 0.000 000 4 = **0.012 mg a.i./kg bw/day** In the guideline exposure scenario, the exposure is 24% of the TSD. In the lax standard scenario, the predicted exposure is 64% of the TSD. • Acute (maximal daily) exposure Lax standard scenario: $Inhalation_{dose}$ + Dermal contact with $surfaces_{dose}$ + Contamination of $fingers_{dose}$ = 0.019 + 0.000 000 6 + 0.032 = **0.051 mg a.i./kg bw** Guideline scenario: $Inhalation_{dose}$ + Dermal contact with $surfaces_{dose}$ = 0.019 + 0.000 000 6 = **0.019 mg a.i./kg bw** In the guideline exposure scenario, the exposure is less than 2% of the TSD_{AC}. In the lax standard scenario, the predicted exposure is less than 4% of the TSD_{AC}. *Predicted doses for passengers from indirect exposure* In this scenario passengers were not present when spraying was carried out and they are exposed through touching surfaces contaminated with spray deposit: for adult passengers **0.000 000 2 mg a.i./kg bw per day (chronic)** **0.000 001 4 mg a.i./kg bw (acute)** for children **0.000 000 02 mg a.i./kg bw per day (chronic)** **0.000 001 8 mg a.i./kg bw (acute)** for toddlers **0.000 000 07 mg a.i./kg bw per day (chronic)** **0.000 005 mg a.i./kg bw (acute)** In all cases these exposures are considered to be acceptable because the predicted doses are well below the TSD or TSD_{AC} (less than 1%).

Generic risk assessment model	Space spray aerosol products for cabin disinsection (permethrin)
	Predicted doses for passengers from direct exposure In this scenario passengers are present when spraying is carried out and they are exposed through inhalation and also through direct skin contact with the spray while spraying is taking place: for adult passengers $Inhalation_{dose}$ + Skin contact with $spray_{dose}$ = 0.000 93 + 0.000 002 = **0.000 93 mg a.i./kg bw per day (chronic)** This is less than 2% of the TSD. $Inhalation_{dose}$ + Skin contact with $spray_{dose}$ = 0.008 5 + 0.000 017 = **0.008 5 mg a.i./kg bw (acute)** for children $Inhalation_{dose}$ + Skin contact with $spray_{dose}$ = 0.000 21 + 0.000 000 4 = **0.000 21 mg a.i./kg bw per day (chronic)** This is less than 1% of the TSD. $Inhalation_{dose}$ + Skin contact with $spray_{dose}$ = 0.016 + 0.000 026 = **0.016 mg a.i./kg bw (acute)** for toddlers $Inhalation_{dose}$ + Skin contact with $spray_{dose}$ = 0.000 51 + 0.000 000 5 = **0.000 51 mg a.i./kg bw per day (chronic)** This is 1% of the TSD. $Inhalation_{dose}$ + Skin contact with $spray_{dose}$ = 0.038 + 0.000 034 = **0.038 mg a.i./kg bw (acute)** For infants $Inhalation_{dose}$ = **0.0011 mg a.i./kg bw per day (chronic)** = **0.077 mg a.i./kg bw (acute)** Exposure of newborn infants is less than 3% of the TSD on a chronic basis. *Assessment* Occupational exposures (cabin crew) are well below the TSD and TSD_{AC} for chronic and acute exposure, respectively.

Generic risk assessment model	Space spray aerosol products for cabin disinsection (permethrin)
	For passengers, exposures from indirect or direct exposure to spray on a chronic basis are less than 3% of the TSD in all cases. Acute exposures are equal to or less than 5% of the TSD_{AC}.

EVALUATION OF RESIDUAL SPRAY CONCENTRATE PRODUCTS (ETOFENPROX)

Product type: Residual spray containing etofenprox for application by ground crew.

Product details: This type of product has been proposed for use, but not yet fully developed and marketed. This evaluation has been conducted on the assumption that the product will be similar to residual spray products containing permethrin. The following parameters are assumed:

- supplied as emulsifiable concentrate formulation (50%), to be diluted to 2% etofenprox for use
- application rate is 0.2 grams etofenprox/m^2 for internal surfaces (0.5 grams/m^2 for floors).

Evaluation of formulation components: Final details of formulation components are not available. Products with a similar formulation composition to residual permethrin products would not be expected to present a particular concern for human health.

Assessment against WHO criteria: Not applicable at this time – the products are still under development.

Alternative presentations of this product type: As with residual products containing permethrin, it is possible that his type of product could also be supplied as a ready-to-use formulation, or applied via a semi-automated fogging device. The following evaluation would also cover such alternatives on a 'worst-case' basis.

Generic risk assessment model	Residual spray concentrate product (etofenprox)
1. Toxicity data Aim: To assess available toxicity data and derive acceptable exposure levels.	**1. Toxicity data** Aim: To assess available toxicity data and derive acceptable exposure levels.
1.1 Conduct literature search for human, animal and in vitro toxicity data and any necessary physicochemical data on the insecticide.	1.1 Literature search on etofenprox conducted on WHO IPCS reviews, JMPR, ATSDR & EFSA.

Generic risk assessment model	Residual spray concentrate product (etofenprox)
1.2 Obtain relevant reviews and key original paper.	1.2 Comprehensive reviews available from IPCS (WHO, 2005), JMPR (JMPR, 1993) and EFSA (EFSA, 2008).
1.3 Tabulate types of study, toxic effects observed, NOAELs and LOAELs.	1.3 All key animal studies tabulated.
1.4 Assess whether quality of database is adequate for risk assessment (range of studies, conduct of studies, adequacy of dose–response data, etc.).	1.4 Studies available on all relevant types of toxicity, most via oral route, with some inhalation and dermal studies. Most conducted to acceptable standards with adequate dose–response data.
1.5 If database is adequate, identify critical toxic effect(s).	1.5 Critical toxic effects in animal tests include hepatic, renal and thyroid changes. No dose response data are available for humans but database from animals is adequate.
1.6 If the insecticide is a skin or respiratory sensitizer, is genotoxic, carcinogenic or extremely acutely toxic, consider whether it is worth proceeding with risk assessment. Consider this also if it produces clear reproductive toxic effects at dose levels causing no general toxicity.	1.6 Etofenprox is not genotoxic, and has not shown carcinogenic or specific reproductive toxic effects. Skin sensitization tests have been negative and no cases of skin or respiratory tract sensitization are reported in the scientific literature. Etofenprox has low acute toxicity and is not irritating to eyes or skin. Toxicokinetic data suggest good or moderate oral absorption (100% oral absorption is assumed in this assessment). Data show 30% dermal absorption. Proceed with risk assessment.
1.7 If 1.6 does not apply, identify pivotal study/studies giving dose–response data for critical effect(s).	1.7 Pivotal studies are: – 2-year rat oral study – 2-year mouse oral study – rabbit developmental toxicity study (treatment on days 6–28 of gestation)
1.8 Identify critical NOAEL(s) from pivotal studies for acute exposure and for longer-term (repeat-dose) exposure.	1.8 Critical NOAELs are: – 2-year oral study, rat, NOAEL = 3.7 mg/kg bw per day – 2-year oral study, mouse, NOAEL= 3.1 mg/kg bw per day – rabbit developmental study, NOAEL = 100 mg/kg bw

Generic risk assessment model	Residual spray concentrate product (etofenprox)
1.9 Assess whether the database allows the setting of TSDs for short-term and long-term exposures.	1.9 Database adequate to allow setting of TSD for single and repeated exposures.
1.10 Set TSDs for oral, dermal or inhalation exposure by dividing NOAEL for the critical effect from the pivotal study via that route by an uncertainty factor (UF): TSD = NOAEL/UF (correcting for systemic bioavailability if necessary). A default UF of 100 is recommended for NOAELs derived from animal studies and 10 for NOAELs derived from human studies.	1.10 The ADI of 0.03 mg/kg bw per day is set by JMPR (JMPR, 1993). This is based on a long-term mouse study with an NOAEL of 3.1 mg/kg bw per day, supported by a long-term rat study with a similar NOAEL (3.7 mg/kg bw per day). Application of a UF of 100 to the lowest NOAEL, 3.1 mg/kg bw per day, results in a TSD of 0.03 mg/kg bw per day. EFSA has set an ARfD of 1.0 mg/kg bw (EFSA, 2008). This is based on a rabbit developmental toxicity study in which an NOAEL of 100 mg/kg bw was identified, with the application of a UF of 100.
1.11 Conclusion on final TSD(s).	1.11 TSDs used in risk characterization: – long-term TSD, 0.03 mg/kg bw per day – short-term TSD_{AC}, 1.0 mg/kg bw
2. Exposure assessment *Aim:* – to estimate occupational exposure via dermal and inhalation routes during mixing, loading and application of residual sprays in an aircraft for disinsection purposes; – to estimate exposure of adult and child passengers (post-application	**2. Exposure assessment: residual product** An emulsifiable concentrate formulation of etofenprox is to be applied to residual spraying. Product only used as a surface spray. The concentration of a.i. in the formulation as supplied is 50%, which is diluted with water to 2% a.i. for the spray solution. The target concentration on surfaces is 0.2 g permethrin/m^2 for interior surfaces and 0.4–0.5 g permethrin/m^2 for floors (essentially the floor is treated twice with the spray solution). The application rate of spray solution is 10 ml/m^2.

Generic risk assessment model	Residual spray concentrate product (etofenprox)
inhalation and dermal exposure, and toddlers' hand-to-mouth exposure). 30% is used for dermal absorption (as derived by EFSA, 2008) 100% default is used for inhalation and gastrointestinal absorption Protection factor of adequate protective equipment, including gloves, is assumed to be 90%. Body weight is 62 kg for adults, 32 kg for older children and 14 kg for toddlers.	[*The above parameters are assumed for this proposed product by analogy with permethrin residual products.*] The guideline scenarios represent a situation where label instructions are being followed. In the lax standard scenarios, it may be assumed, for example, that no gloves are used or that spraying equipment is not totally leakproof.
2.1 Ground crew operator exposure *a) Mixing and loading* In mixing and loading, only dermal exposure is considered significant. It is assumed that the amount of the spray liquid prepared per day to treat the interior surfaces of a large aircraft is three 10-litre tanks. The floors are treated twice. For the purposes of the calculations the floor area is assumed to be one-third of the interior surface. This requires an additional 10-litre tank. It is also assumed that ground personnel need to spray an aeroplane twice a week throughout the year.	**2.1 Ground crew operator exposure** *a) Mixing and loading* Product used is a 2% emulsion, diluted from 50% a.i. by ground staff or authorised applicators. Chronic systemic dose due to dermal exposure, mg a.i./kg bw per day: 0.04 ml × 500 mg a.i./ml × 1.0 × 30% × 104 days/(62 kg × 365 days) = **0.028 mg a.i./kg bw per day** (lax standard scenario) In guideline scenario calculation, a protection factor of 90% applies, hence the systemic dose is: 0.04 ml × 500 mg a.i./ml × 0.1 × 30% × 104 days/(62 kg × 365 days) = **0.0028 mg a.i./kg bw per day** The maximum daily systemic dose will be: 0.04 ml × 500 mg a.i./ml × 1.0 × 30%/62 kg = **0.097 mg/kg bw** (lax standard scenario)

Generic risk assessment model	Residual spray concentrate product (etofenprox)
In the guideline scenario, gloves are used. In the lax standard scenario, no gloves are assumed. Default values for hand contamination while mixing and loading are available (0.01 ml/operation).	0.04 ml × 500 mg a.i./ml × 0.1 × 30%/62 kg = **0.0097 mg/kg bw** (guideline scenario)
b) Application The quantity of spray to be applied depends on the area of the internal surfaces of the aircraft. A large aircraft with an internal surface area of 2500 m^2 and a volume of 1000 m^3 is assumed for these calculations. The required dosage is 0.2 g a.i./m^2 for interior surfaces and 0.4–0.5 g a.i./m^2 for floors. With the 2% preparation, 10 ml of the spray liquid must be applied per square metre. With a sprayer adjusted to deliver 1 ml/s, the correct deposit will be achieved if one square metre is sprayed per second. The floors are treated twice. It is assumed, that 9.3 ml of spray liquid will contaminate hands during one work day. Breathing rate 1.9 m^3/hour, work time 2 hours – air volume inhaled = 3.8 m^3. It is assumed that 0.1% of the a.i. sprayed will be	*b) Application* As the spray liquid is 2% emulsion, the spray concentration will be 20 mg/ml. Concentration of the aerosol in the inhaled air: 10 ml of spray is applied/m^2, which in a large aircraft means that 25 litres, or 25 000 ml, of spray liquid is needed. Approximately 0.1% of the sprayed a.i. is assumed to be evenly distributed in the air, i.e. in a volume of 1000 m^3. The inhalable concentration (CA) of the aerosol would then be 0.001 × 25000/1000 ml/m^3 = 0.025 ml of spray/m^3. Systemic dose due to inhalation exposure, mg a.i./kg bw per day: 20 mg/ml × 0.025 ml/m^3 × 1.0 × 3.8 m^3 × 100% × 104 days/(62 kg × 365 days) = **0.0087 mg a.i./kg bw per day** (lax standard scenario) In the guideline scenario, the use of protective equipment provides a 90% protection factor. The exposure will therefore be 10% of that in the lax standard scenario, i.e. **0.00087 mg a.i./kg bw per day** The maximum daily systemic dose will be: 20 mg/ml × 0.025 ml/m^3 × 1.0 × 3.8 m^3 × 100%/62 = **0.031 mg a.i./kg bw** (lax standard scenario 20 mg/ml × 0.025 ml/m^3 × 0.1 × 3.8 m^3 × 100%/62 = **0.0031 mg a.i./kg bw** (guideline scenario) Systemic dose due to dermal exposure, mg a.i./kg bw per day:

Generic risk assessment model	Residual spray concentrate product (etofenprox)
evenly distributed in the air (including in the breathing zone of the operator). The default absorption rate from the respiratory tract is 100%.	9.3 ml/day × 20 mg/ml × 1.0 × 30% × 104 days/(62 kg × 365 days) = **0.26 mg a.i./kg bw per day** (lax standard scenario) In the guideline scenario calculation, the protection factor for protective clothing (90%) is applied, and the systemic dose is **0.026 mg a.i./kg bw per day** The maximum daily systemic dose will be: 9.3 ml/day × 20 mg/ml × 1.0 × 30%/62 kg = **0.9 mg a.i./kg bw** (lax standard scenario) 9.3 ml/day × 20 mg/ml × 0.1 × 30%/62 kg = **0.09 mg a.i./kg bw** (guideline scenario)
2.2 Cabin crew and passenger exposure from residual disinsection Passenger and cabin crew exposure is assumed to be due to secondary dermal exposure from contact with the surfaces of the aircraft. For passengers and cabin crew, the proportion translodged onto bare skin is 11%; the exposed area of skin reflects the clothing worn, with an additional component for toddlers because of greater activity. For cabin crew, the exposed skin area is 0.1 m^2 (50% of hands and forearms) and the exposure duration is 240 days per year. For passengers, the exposed skin areas are 0.25 m^2 for adults, 0.16 m^2 for older children, and 0.2 m^2 for toddlers. Exposure duration is 40 days	**2.2 Cabin crew and passenger exposure from residual disinsection** Product specific target concentration on the surfaces, 0.2 g/m^2 = 200 mg/m^2. The higher dose applied to floors is balanced by lower transfer from carpet to skin (USEPA, 2009), hence all calculations can be based on 0.2 g/m^2. Systemic dose of cabin crew members due to dermal exposure, mg a.i./kg bw per day: 200 mg/m^2 × 11% × 0.1 m^2 × 30% × 240 days/(62 kg × 365 days) = **0.007 mg a.i./kg bw per day** Maximum daily exposure: 200 mg/m^2 × 11% × 0.1 m^2 × 30%/62 kg = **0.01 mg a.i./kg bw.** Systemic dose of the passengers due to dermal exposure, mg a.i./kg bw per day: 200 mg/m^2 × 11% × (0.25 m^2, 0.16 m^2 or 0.2 m^2) × 30% × (40 days or 5 days)/((62 kg, 32 kg or 14 kg) × 365 days) Long-term exposures: for adults: **0.003 mg a.i./kg bw per day** for children: **0.00045 mg a.i./kg bw per day** for toddlers: **0.0013 mg a.i./kg bw per day** Maximum daily exposures: for adults: **0.026 mg a.i./kg bw**

Generic risk assessment model	Residual spray concentrate product (etofenprox)
for adult passengers and 5 days for children. In addition, the sprayed insecticide may be dislodged from surfaces as contaminated dust leading to ingestion by toddlers due to hand-to-mouth behaviour. For estimating the hand-to-mouth exposure, the relevant hand area for toddlers is 0.032 m^2. For the extent of the transfer from hands to mouth, a default of 10% is used.	for children: **0.033 mg a.i./kg bw** for toddlers: **0.094 mg a.i./kg bw** Systemic dose due to hand-to-mouth behaviour, toddlers, mg a.i./kg bw per day: 200 mg/m^2 × 11% × 0.032 m^2 × 10% × 100% × 5 days/(14 kg × 365 days) = **0.00007 mg a.i./kg bw per day** Maximum daily exposure: 200 mg/m^2 × 11% × 0.032 m^2 × 10% × 100%/14 kg = **0.005 mg a.i./kg bw**
3. Risk characterization 3.1 Compare exposure estimates with TSDs for risk characterization. For products with appreciable acute toxicity, comparison against TSD_{AC} should also be considered. 3.2 If the exposure calculated for a subgroup and exposure route is below the respective TSD, using conservative estimates, it can be assumed that the exposure is acceptable and does not cause unacceptable risk to human health. 3.3 If the exposure is above the TSD and refining the assessment process, e.g. by use of chemical-specific data, fails to bring the exposure below the TSD,	**3. Risk characterization** Etofenprox has low acute toxicity. The risk assessment is based on:- – comparison of chronic exposure with the long-term TSD; – comparison of acute exposure with the short-term TSD_{AC}. From section 1.10, the TSD used in long-term risk characterization is 0.03 mg/kg bw per day. Short-term guidance value (TSD_{AC}) is 1.0 mg/kg bw. **Predicted doses to be used in subsequent risk characterization:** *Total operator predicted dose, ground personnel performing residual disinsections:* • Long-term (TWA) exposure Lax standard scenario: $dose_{M/L}$ dermal + $dose_A$ inhalation + $dose_A$ dermal = 0.028 + 0.0087 + 0.26

Generic risk assessment model	Residual spray concentrate product (etofenprox)
measures to reduce the exposure must be implemented. 3.4 In some cases the exposure may be found to be unacceptable, despite measures to reduce it. Other methods of vector control should be considered.	= **0.3 mg a.i./kg bw per day** Guideline scenario: $dose_{M/L}$ dermal + $dose_A$ inhalation + $dose_A$ dermal = 0.0028 + 0.00087 + 0.026 = **0.03 mg a.i./kg bw per day** where: $dose_{M/L}$ refers to exposure from mixing and loading, and $dose_A$ refers to exposure from application In the guideline exposure scenario, the total predicted dose is equal to the TSD. In the lax standard scenario, the TSD may be exceeded by a factor of 10. It is therefore important to make sure that safe practices are implemented, that adequate PPE is used, and that the equipment is maintained in good working condition. • Acute (maximal daily) exposure Lax standard scenario: $dose_{M/L}$ dermal + $dose_A$ inhalation + $dose_A$ dermal = 0.097 + 0.031 + 0.9 = **1.03 mg a.i./kg bw** Guideline scenario: $dose_{M/L}$ dermal + $dose_A$ inhalation + $dose_A$ dermal = 0.0097 + 0.0031 + 0.09 = **0.103 mg a.i./kg bw** In the guideline exposure scenario the maximal daily dose is approximately 10% of the TSD_{AC}. In the lax standard scenario, acute worker exposure is approximately equal to the TSD_{AC}. It is therefore important to make sure that safe practices are implemented, that adequate PPE is used, and that the equipment is maintained in good working condition. *Total cabin crew predicted dose:* Dose from touching contaminated surfaces = **0.007 mg a.i./kg bw per day (TWA) or 0.01 mg a.i./kg bw (maximal daily exposure)**

Generic risk assessment model	Residual spray concentrate product (etofenprox)
	Cabin crew exposure is considered to be acceptable. The predicted doses are 23% of the TSD and 1% of the TSD_{AC}. *Total passenger predicted doses:* • Long-term exposure: for adult passengers **0.003 mg a.i./kg bw per day** for children **0.00045 mg a.i./kg bw per day** • Maximum daily exposures: for adult passengers **0.026 mg a.i./kg bw** for children **0.033 mg a.i./kg bw** Exposure of adult and child passengers from residual treatment is considered to be acceptable – the predicted doses are between 1% and 10% of the TSD and less than 4% of the TSD_{AC}. *Total passenger predicted doses – toddlers:* • Long-term dose from touching contaminated surfaces + dose from hand-to-mouth behaviour = 0.0013 + 0.00007 = **0.0014 mg a.i./kg bw per day** • Maximum daily exposure from touching contaminated surfaces + dose from hand-to-mouth behaviour = 0.094 + 0.005 = **0.1 mg a.i./kg bw** Exposure of toddlers from residual treatment is considered to be acceptable – the predicted doses represent 5% and 10% of the TSD and TSD_{AC}, respectively.

EVALUATION OF SPACE SPRAY AEROSOL PRODUCTS FOR CABIN DISINSECTION (ETOFENPROX)

Product type: Aerosol spray can product containing etofenprox for space spraying by cabin crew.

Product details: This type of product has been proposed for use, but not yet fully developed and marketed. This evaluation has been conducted on the assumption that the use rates of the product will be similar to existing space spray disinsection products containing d-phenothrin or permethrin (35 grams of formulation per 100 cubic metres). An aerosol spray can containing 0.7% etofenprox is proposed.

Evaluation of formulation components: Final details of formulation components are not available. Products with a similar formulation composition to existing space spray aircraft disinsection products would not be expected to present a particular concern for human health.

Assessment against WHO criteria: Not applicable at this time – the products are still under development.

Generic risk assessment model	Space spray aerosol products for cabin disinsection (etofenprox)
1. Toxicity data	**1. Toxicity data**
Aim: To assess available toxicity data and derive acceptable exposure levels	Aim: To assess available toxicity data and derive acceptable exposure levels
1.1 Conduct literature search for human, animal and in vitro toxicity data and any necessary physicochemical data on the insecticide	1.1 Literature search on etofenprox conducted on WHO IPCS reviews, JMPR, ATSDR & EFSA.
1.2 Obtain relevant reviews and key original papers	1.2 Comprehensive reviews available from IPCS (WHO, 2005), JMPR (JMPR, 1993) and EFSA (2008)
1.3 Tabulate types of study, toxic effects observed, NOAELs and LOAELs.	1.3 All key animal studies tabulated.

Generic risk assessment model	Space spray aerosol products for cabin disinsection (etofenprox)
1.4 Assess whether quality of database is adequate for risk assessment (range of studies, conduct of studies, adequacy of dose–response data, etc.).	1.4 Studies available on all relevant types of toxicity, most via oral route, with some inhalation and dermal studies. Most conducted to acceptable standards with adequate dose–response data.
1.5 If database is adequate, identify critical toxic effect(s).	1.5 Critical toxic effects in animal tests include hepatic, renal and thyroid changes. No dose response data are available for humans but database from animals is adequate.
1.6 If the insecticide is a skin or respiratory sensitizer, is genotoxic, carcinogenic or extremely acutely toxic, consider whether it is worth proceeding with risk assessment. Consider this also if it produces clear reproductive toxic effects at dose levels causing no general toxicity.	1.6 Etofenprox is not genotoxic, and has not shown carcinogenic or specific reproductive toxic effects. Skin sensitization tests have been negative and no cases of skin or respiratory tract sensitization are reported in the scientific literature. Etofenprox has low acute toxicity and is not irritating to eyes or skin. Toxicokinetic data suggest good or moderate oral absorption (100% oral absorption is assumed in this assessment). Data show 30% dermal absorption. Proceed with risk assessment.
1.7 If 1.6 does not apply, identify pivotal study/studies giving dose–response data for critical effect(s).	1.7 Pivotal studies are: – 2-year rat oral study – 2-year mouse oral study – rabbit developmental toxicity study (treatment on days 6–28 of gestation)
1.8 Identify critical NOAEL(s) from pivotal studies for acute exposure and for longer-term (repeat-dose) exposure.	1.8 Critical NOAELs are: – 2-year oral study, rat, NOAEL = 3.7 mg/kg bw per day – 2-year oral study, mouse, NOAEL= 3.1 mg/kg bw per day – rabbit developmental study, NOAEL = 100 mg/kg bw
1.9 Assess whether the database allows the setting of TSDs for short-term and long-term exposures.	1.9 Database adequate to allow setting of TSD for single and repeated exposures.

Generic risk assessment model	Space spray aerosol products for cabin disinsection (etofenprox)
1.10 Set TSDs for oral, dermal or inhalation exposure by dividing NOAEL for the critical effect from the pivotal study via that route by an uncertainty factor (UF): TSD = NOAEL/UF (correcting for systemic bioavailability if necessary). A default UF of 100 is recommended for NOAELs derived from animal studies and 10 for NOAELs derived from human studies.	1.10 The ADI of 0.03 mg/kg bw per day is set by JMPR (JMPR, 1993). This is based on a long-term mouse study with an NOAEL of 3.1 mg/kg bw per day, supported by a long-term rat study with a similar NOAEL (3.7 mg/kg bw per day). Application of a UF of 100 to the lowest NOAEL, 3.1 mg/kg bw per day, results in a TSD of 0.03 mg/kg bw per day. EFSA has set an ARfD of 1.0 mg/kg bw (EFSA, 2008). This is based on a rabbit developmental toxicity study in which an NOAEL of 100 mg/kg bw was identified, with the application of a UF of 100.
1.11 Conclusion on final TSD(s).	1.11 TSDs used in risk characterization: – long-term TSD, 0.03 mg/kg bw per day – short-term TSD_{AC}, 1.0 mg/kg bw
2. Exposure assessment *Aim:* – to estimate occupational exposure via dermal and inhalation routes resulting from spraying aerosol sprays in an aircraft for disinsection purposes; – to estimate exposure of adult and child passengers (post-application inhalation and dermal exposure, and toddlers' hand-to-mouth exposure).	**2. Exposure assessment: aerosol spray product** An aerosol product containing 0.7% etofenprox for space spraying, packed in an aerosol can with a propellant. Spray rate (discharge rate from can) is 0.8–1.2 g/s. For the purposes of this risk assessment a large aircraft (volume 1000 m^3) is assumed, with a scenario of four 100 g cans being discharged. The guideline scenarios represent a situation where label instructions are being followed and assume that the products used are in good working order Touching surfaces is the only source of dermal exposure in the guideline scenario. In the lax standard scenario the spray nozzle may leak leading to fingers becoming contaminated.

Generic risk assessment model	Space spray aerosol products for cabin disinsection (etofenprox)
30% is used for dermal absorption (as derived by EFSA, 2008) 100% default is used for inhalation and gastrointestinal absorption Body weight is 62 kg for adults, 32 kg for older children and 14 kg for toddlers.	
2.1 Space spraying, cabin crew exposure, application Default values for the general exposure parameters needed for inhalation exposure assessment with ConsExpo software are: – the spray duration (in this case estimated 200 seconds); – exposure duration (30 minutes); – room volume (or in this case, volume of the cabin, large aircraft, default 1000 m^3); – room height (estimated 2 m); – ventilation rate (as a worst case it is assumed that there is no effect due to ventilation). The remaining parameters needed for the software are product-specific.	***2.1 Space spraying, cabin crew exposure, application*** The product specific parameters required by the ConsExpo inhalation model are: – the mass generation rate, or the amount of compound released from the can during spraying per unit of time (2 g/s to reflect two cans being discharged simultaneously in this example scenario); – estimate of the airborne, non-volatile fraction (a worst-case assumption has been made, that this fraction is 100%); – inhalation cut-off droplet diameter (15 μm); – weight fraction of non-volatiles (default 2%); – weight fraction of compound of interest in the product (percentage of a.i. in the product, 0.7%); – density of non-volatile compounds (assumed 1.8 g/cm^3); – initial particle distribution (assumed log-normal, average particle diameter 8 μm, coefficient of variation 0.45). *Systemic dose due to inhalation exposure*: These exposure estimates are obtained directly from the output of the ConsExpo software. **0.0056 mg a.i./kg bw per day** (ConsExpo Output – inhalation chronic systemic dose, point-estimate)

Generic risk assessment model	Space spray aerosol products for cabin disinsection (etofenprox)
Respiration rate of cabin crew members is assumed to be 0.89 m^3/h. Space spray is not intended to settle on surfaces, but is likely to be carried away by the air circulation. It can be assumed that 1% of the material sprayed into the air could be deposited on the surfaces. If four 100 g cans are discharged (400 g spray), containing 0.7% a.i. (2.8 g), into a large aircraft with a surface area of 2500 m^2, then the amount which settles would be (2.8 g × 1%)/2500 m^2 = 0.011 mg/m^2.	**0.0085 mg a.i./kg bw per day** (ConsExpo Output – inhalation acute systemic dose, point-estimate) *Systemic dose due to dermal exposure via body areas in contact with surfaces:* 0.011 mg/m^2 × 11% × 0.1 m^2 × 240 days × 30%/62 kg × 365 days = **0.000 000 4 mg a.i./kg bw per day** *Systemic dose due to dermal exposure via contamination of fingers with spray liquid (leaking nozzle):* 1 ml/day × 7 mg/ml × 240 days × 30%/62 kg × 365 days =**0.022 mg a.i./kg bw per day** For guideline scenario, systemic dose due to dermal exposure = contact with surfaces only = **0.000 000 4 mg a.i./kg bw per day** For lax standard scenario, systemic dose due to dermal exposure = contact with surfaces + contamination of fingers = 0.000 000 4 + 0.022 = **0.022 mg a.i./kg bw per day** • Maximum daily exposures from body areas in contact with surfaces: 0.011 mg/m^2 × 11% × 0.1 m^2 × 30%/62 kg = **0.000 000 6 mg a.i./kg bw** • Maximum daily exposures from contamination of fingers: 1 ml/day × 7 mg/ml × 30%/62 kg = **0.034 mg a.i./kg bw** For guideline scenario, maximum daily exposure is: **0.000 000 6 mg a.i./kg bw** For lax standard scenario, maximum daily exposure is: 0.000 000 6 + 0.034 = **0.034 mg a.i./kg bw**

Generic risk assessment model	Space spray aerosol products for cabin disinsection (etofenprox)
2.2 Space spraying, passenger exposure For the systemic dose due to indirect dermal exposure (to material deposited on surfaces), exposed skin areas are 0.25 m^2 for adults, 0.16 m^2 for older children, 0.2 m^2 for toddlers. The material deposited on surfaces is calculated in the same way as for cabin crew. If passengers are present during space spraying, the pattern of inhalation exposure is considered to be similar to crew members' exposure. Exposure frequencies are 40 days/year for adult passengers and 5 days/year for children of all ages. See model parameters used in cabin crew exposure calculations. Breathing rates (resting rates) for adult passengers are 0.40 m^3/h, for children 6–11 years and toddlers 0.38 m^3/h, and for newborn infants 0.28 m^3/h. For the systemic dose due to direct dermal contact with the spray, exposed skin areas are 0.33 m^2 for adults, 0.26 m^2 for older children, and 0.15 m^2 for toddlers (based on the head and half of the hands, forearms and lower legs).	***2.2 Space spraying, passenger exposure*** *Systemic dose due to indirect dermal exposure (passengers not present during space spraying – body areas in contact with surfaces where material has deposited):* 0.011 mg/m^2 × 11% × (0.25, 0.16 or 0.2 m^2) × (40 or 5 days) × 30%/(62, 32 or 14 kg) × 365 days (chronic exposure) for adult passengers **0.000 000 2 mg a.i./kg bw per day** for children **0.000 000 032 mg a.i./kg bw per day** for toddlers **0.000 000 07 mg a.i./kg bw per day** • Maximal daily exposure 0.011 mg/m^2 × 11% × (0.25, 0.16 or 0.2 m^2) × 30%/(62, 32 or 14 kg) for adult passengers **0.000 001 5 mg a.i./kg bw** for children **0.000 001 8 mg a.i./kg bw** for toddlers **0.000 005 mg a.i./kg bw** *Systemic dose due to inhalation exposure (passengers present during space spraying):* The exposure estimates are obtained directly from the output of the ConsExpo software. The underlying algorithms are not shown in this worked example: for adult passengers **0.0004 mg a.i./kg bw per day (chronic)** **0.0038 mg a.i./kg bw (acute)** for children **0.0001 mg a.i./kg bw per day (chronic)** **0.007 mg a.i./kg bw (acute)** for toddlers **0.0002 mg a.i./kg bw per day (chronic)** **0.017 mg a.i./kg bw (acute)**

Generic risk assessment model	Space spray aerosol products for cabin disinsection (etofenprox)
For newborn infants, only inhalation exposure is considered to be relevant because infants will be held or transported in their own carriers and will have very limited opportunity for contact with aircraft surfaces	for newborn infants **0.0005 mg a.i./kg bw per day (chronic)** **0.034 mg a.i./kg bw (acute)** (ConsExpo Output – inhalation systemic doses, point-estimates) *Systemic dose due to direct skin contact with the spray (passengers present during space spraying:* 0.011 mg/m^2 × (0.33, 0.26 or 0.15 m^2) × (40 or 5 days) × 30%/(62, 32 or 14 kg) × 365 days (chronic exposure) for adult passengers **0.000 002 mg a.i./kg bw per day** for children **0.000 000 4 mg a.i./kg bw per day** for toddlers **0.000 000 5 mg a.i./kg bw per day** • Maximal daily exposure 0.011 mg/m^2 × (0.33, 0.26 or 0.15 m^2) × 30%/(62, 32 or 14 kg) for adult passengers **0.000 04 mg a.i./kg bw** for children **0.000 03 mg a.i./kg bw** for toddlers **0.000 04 mg a.i./kg bw**
3. Risk characterization	***3. Risk characterization***
3.1 Compare exposure estimates with TSDs for risk characterization. For products with appreciable acute toxicity, consideration should be given to comparing against TSD_{AC}. 3.2 If the exposure calculated for a subgroup and exposure route is below the respective TSD,	The risk assessment is based on: – comparison of chronic exposure with the long-term TSD; – comparison of acute exposure with the short-term TSD_{AC}. From section 1.10, the TSD used in long-term risk characterization is 0.03 mg/kg bw per day for etofenprox. Short-term guidance value (TSD_{AC}) is 1.0 mg/kg bw.

Generic risk assessment model	Space spray aerosol products for cabin disinsection (etofenprox)
using conservative estimates, it can be assumed that the exposure is acceptable and does not cause unacceptable risk to human health. 3.3 If the exposure is above the TSD and refining the assessment process, e.g. by use of chemical-specific data, fails to bring the exposure below the TSD, measures to reduce the exposure must be implemented. 3.4 In some cases the exposure may be found to be unacceptable despite measures to reduce it. Other methods of vector control should be considered.	***Predicted doses to be used in subsequent risk characterization:*** *Total predicted dose, cabin crew performing space spraying:* • Long-term (TWA) exposure Lax standard scenario: $Inhalation_{dose}$ + Dermal contact with $surfaces_{dose}$ + Contamination of $fingers_{dose}$ = 0.0056 + 0.000 000 4 + 0.022 = **0.028 mg a.i./kg bw per day** Guideline scenario: $Inhalation_{dose}$ + Dermal contact with $surfaces_{dose}$ = 0.0056 + 0.000 000 4 = **0.0056 mg a.i./kg bw/day** In the guideline exposure scenario, the exposure is 19% of the TSD. In the lax standard scenario, the predicted exposure is 93% of the TSD. • Acute (maximal daily) exposure Lax standard scenario: $Inhalation_{dose}$ + Dermal contact with $surfaces_{dose}$ + Contamination of $fingers_{dose}$ = 0.0085 + 0.000 000 6 + 0.034 = **0.043 mg a.i./kg bw** Guideline scenario: $Inhalation_{dose}$ + Dermal contact with $surfaces_{dose}$ = 0.0085 + 0.000 000 6 = **0.0085 mg a.i./kg bw** In the guideline exposure scenario, the exposure is less than 1% of the TSD_{AC}. In the lax standard scenario, the predicted exposure is less than 5% of the TSD_{AC}. *Predicted doses for passengers from indirect exposure* In this scenario passengers were not present when spraying was carried out and they are exposed through touching surfaces contaminated with spray deposit: for adult passengers **0.000 000 2 mg a.i./kg bw per day (chronic)** **0.000 001 5 mg a.i./kg bw (acute)**

Generic risk assessment model	Space spray aerosol products for cabin disinsection (etofenprox)
	for children **0.000 000 032 mg a.i./kg bw per day (chronic)** **0.000 001 8 mg a.i./kg bw (acute)** for toddlers **0.000 000 07 mg a.i./kg bw per day (chronic)** **0.000 005 mg a.i./kg bw (acute)** In all cases these exposures are considered to be acceptable because the predicted doses are well below the TSD or TSD_{AC} (less than 1%). *Predicted doses for passengers from direct exposure* In this scenario passengers are present when spraying is carried out and they are exposed through inhalation and also through direct skin contact with the spray while spraying is taking place: for adult passengers $Inhalation_{dose}$ + Skin contact with $spray_{dose}$ = 0.000 4 + 0.000 002 = **0.000 4 mg a.i./kg bw per day (chronic)** This is less than 2% of the TSD. $Inhalation_{dose}$ + Skin contact with $spray_{dose}$ = 0.003 8 + 0.000 04 = **0.003 8 mg a.i./kg bw (acute)** for children $Inhalation_{dose}$ + Skin contact with $spray_{dose}$ = 0.000 1 + 0.000 000 4 = **0.000 1 mg a.i./kg bw per day (chronic)** This is less than 1% of the TSD. $Inhalation_{dose}$ + Skin contact with $spray_{dose}$ = 0.007 + 0.000 03 = **0.007 mg a.i./kg bw (acute)** for toddlers $Inhalation_{dose}$ + Skin contact with $spray_{dose}$ = 0.000 2 + 0.000 000 5 = **0.000 2 mg a.i./kg bw per day (chronic)** This is less than 1% of the TSD. $Inhalation_{dose}$ + Skin contact with $spray_{dose}$

Generic risk assessment model	Space spray aerosol products for cabin disinsection (etofenprox)
	= 0.017 + 0.000 04 = **0.017 mg a.i./kg bw (acute)** For infants $Inhalation_{dose}$ = **0.0005 mg a.i./kg bw per day (chronic)** = **0.034 mg a.i./kg bw (acute)** Exposure of newborn infants is less than 2% of the TSD on a chronic basis. *Assessment* Occupational exposures (cabin crew) on a chronic basis are below the TSD for the guideline and lax standard scenarios, and acute exposures are predicted to be well below the TSD_{AC}. For passengers, exposures from indirect or direct exposure to spray on a chronic basis are less than 2% of the TSD in all cases. Acute exposures are all less than 5% of the TSD_{AC}.

EVALUATION OF OTHER TYPES OF DISINSECTION METHOD

It is noted that other methods for disinsection of aircraft are under development.

Product type: Use of ozone for aircraft disinsection purposes.

Description of the method: The proposed method is to generate an ozone concentration within the aircraft cabin of >10 mg/m^3 in the absence of personnel aboard the aircraft.

Human health risks associated with this method include the direct effects of any residual ozone not purged from the aircraft cabin after treatment, and the effects of chemicals which may be formed in the cabin due to the reaction of ozone with the chemicals and materials present in the aircraft cabin. The Expert Consultation concluded that there were significant potential health concerns associated with the use of ozone but the generic risk assessment model would not be an appropriate method to assess those risks.

REFERENCES

EFSA (2008). Conclusion on the peer review of etofenprox. European Food Safety Authority, Parma, Italy. *EFSA Scientific Report*, **213**: 1–131 (available at: http://www.efsa.europa.eu/en/efsajournal/doc/213r.pdf).

IARC (1991). IARC Monographs on the evaluation of carcinogenic risks to humans. Occupational exposures in insecticide application, and some pesticides (IARC Monographs volume 53). International Agency for Research on Cancer, Lyons, France (available at: http://monographs.iarc.fr/ENG/Monographs/vol53/mono53-13.pdf).

JMPR (1988). Pesticide residues in food – 1988. Report of the Joint Meeting of the FAO Panel of Experts on Pesticide Residues in Food and the Environment and a WHO Expert Group on Pesticide Residues. FAO Plant Production and Protection Paper 92. Food and Agriculture Organization of the United Nations, Rome, Italy.

JMPR (1993). Pesticide residues in food – 1993. Report of the Joint Meeting of the FAO Panel of Experts on Pesticide Residues in Food and the Environment and a WHO Expert Group on Pesticide Residues. FAO Plant Production and Protection Paper 122. Food and Agriculture Organization of the United Nations, Rome, Italy (available at: http://www.fao.org/ag/AGP/AGPP/Pesticid/JMPR/Download/93_rep/Report1993.pdf).

JMPR (1999). Pesticide residues in food – 1999. Report of the Joint Meeting of the FAO Panel of Experts on Pesticide Residues in Food and the Environment and the WHO Core Assessment Group. FAO Plant Production and Protection Paper 153. Food and Agriculture Organization of the United Nations, Rome, Italy (available at: http://www.fao.org/ag/AGP/AGPP/Pesticid/JMPR/Download/99_rep/REPORT1999.pdf).

JMPR (2002). Pesticide residues in food – 2002. Report of the Joint Meeting of the FAO Panel of Experts on Pesticide Residues in Food and the Environment and the WHO Core Assessment Group. FAO Plant Production and Protection Paper 172. Food and Agriculture Organization of the United Nations, Rome, Italy (available at: http://www.fao.org/ag/AGP/AGPP/Pesticid/JMPR/Download/2002_rep/2002JMPRReport2.pdf).

WHO (2005). *Safety of pyrethroids for public health use*. Geneva, World Health Organization, Geneva, Switzerland (WHO/CDS/WHOPES/GCDPP/2005.10; available at: http://whqlibdoc.who.int/hq/2005/WHO_CDS_WHOPES_GCDPP_2005.10.pdf).

Diazinon (No. 198, 1997)
1,2-Dibromoethane(No. 177, 1996)
Di-*n*-butyl phthalate (No. 189, 1997)
1,2-Dichloroethane (No. 62, 1987, 1st edition), (No. 176, 1995, 2nd edition)
2,4-Dichlorophenoxyacetic acid (2,4-D) (No. 29, 1984)
2,4-Dichlorophenoxyacetic acid - environmental aspects (No. 84, 1989)
1 ,3-Dichloropropene, 1,2-dichloropropane and mixtures (No. 146, 1993)
Dichlorvos (No. 79, 1988)
Dinitro-*ortho*-cresol (No. 220, 2000)
Diesel fuel and exhaust emissions (No. 171, 1996)
Diethylhexyl phthalate (No. 131, 1992)
Diflubenzuron (No. 184, 1996)
Dimethoate (No. 90, 1989)
Dimethylformamide (No. 114, 1991)
Dimethyl sulfate (No. 48, 1985)
Diseases of suspected chemical etiology and their prevention, principles of studies on (No. 72, 1987)
Disinfectants and disinfectant by-products (No. 216, 1999)
Dithiocarbamate pesticides, ethylenethiourea, and propylenethiourea: a general introduction (No. 78, 1988)
Dose–response for the risk assessment of chemicals, principles for modelling (No. 239, 2009)
Electromagnetic fields (No. 137, 1992)
Elemental speciation in human health risk assessment (No. 234, 2006)
Endosulfan (No. 40, 1984)
Endrin (No. 130, 1992)
Environmental epidemiology, guidelines on studies in (No. 27, 1983)
Epichlorohydrin (No. 33, 1984)
Essential trace elements: Principles and methods for the assessment of risk (No. 228, 2001)
Ethylbenzene (No. 186, 1996)
Ethylene oxide (No. 55, 1985)
Extremely low frequency (ELF) fields (No. 36, 1984)
Extremely low frequency fields (No. 238, 2007)
Exposure to chemicals, principles for evaluating health risks in children associated with (No. 237, 2006)
Fenitrothion (No. 133, 1992)
Fenvalerate (No. 95, 1990)
Flame retardants: a general introduction (No. 192, 1997)
Flame retardants: tris(chloropropyl) phosphate and tris(2-chloroethyl) phosphate (No. 209, 1998)
Flame retardants: tris(2-butoxyethyl) phosphate, tris(2-ethylhexyl) phosphate and tetrakis(hydroxymethyl) phosphonium salts (No. 218, 2000)
Fluorides (No. 227, 2001)
Fluorine and fluorides (No. 36, 1984)
Food additives and contaminants in food, principles for the safety assessment of (No. 70, 1987)
Formaldehyde (No. 89, 1989)
Fumonisin B1 (No. 219, 2000)
Genetic effects in human populations, guidelines for the study of (No. 46, 1985)
Glyphosate (No. 159, 1994)
Guidance values for human exposure limits (No. 170, 1994)
Heptachlor (No. 38, 1984)
Hexachlorobenzene (No. 195, 1997)
Hexachlorobutadiene (No. 156, 1994)
Alpha- and *beta*-hexachlorocyclohexanes (No. 123, 1992)
Hexachlorocyclopentadiene (No. 120, 1991)
n-Hexane (No. 122, 1991)
Human exposure assessment (No. 214, 2000)
Hydrazine (No. 68, 1987)
Hydrogen sulfide (No. 19, 1981)
Hydroquinone (No. 157, 1994)
Immunotoxicity associated with exposure to chemicals, principles and methods for assessing direct (No. 180, 1996)
Infancy and early childhood, principles for evaluating health risks from chemicals during (No. 59, 1986)
Isobenzan (No. 129, 1991)
Isophorone (No. 174, 1995)
Kelevan (No. 66, 1986)
Lasers and optical radiation (No. 23, 1982)
Lead (No. 3, 1977)
Lead, inorganic (No. 165, 1995)
Lead - environmental aspects (No. 85, 1989)
Lindane (No. 124, 1991)
Linear alkylbenzene sulfonates and related compounds (No. 169, 1996)
Magnetic fields (No. 69, 1987)
Man-made mineral fibres (No. 77, 1988)
Manganese (No. 17, 1981)
Mercury (No.1, 1976)
Mercury - environmental aspects (No. 86, 1989)
Mercury, inorganic (No. 118,1991)
Methanol (No. 196, 1997)
Methomyl (No. 178, 1996)
2-Methoxyethanol, 2-ethoxyethanol, and their acetates (No. 115, 1990)
Methyl bromide (No. 166, 1995)
Methylene chloride (No. 32, 1984, 1st edition), (No. 164, 1996, 2nd edition)

THE ENVIRONMENTAL HEALTH CRITERIA SERIES (continued)

Methyl ethyl ketone (No. 143, 1992)
Methyl isobutyl ketone (No. 117, 1990)
Methylmercury (No. 101, 1990)
Methyl parathion (No. 145, 1992)
Methyl *tertiary*-butyl ether (No. 206, 1998)
Mirex (No. 44, 1984)
Morpholine (No. 179, 1996)
Mutagenic and carcinogenic chemicals, guide to short-term tests for detecting (No. 51, 1985)
Mycotoxins (No. 11, 1979)
Mycotoxins, selected: ochratoxins, trichothecenes, ergot (No. 105, 1990)
Nephrotoxicity associated with exposure to chemicals, principles and methods for the assessment of (No. 119,1991)
Neurotoxicity associated with exposure to chemicals, principles and methods for the assessment of (No. 60, 1986)
Neurotoxicity risk assessment for human health, principles and approaches (No. 223, 2001)
Nickel (No. 108, 1991)
Nitrates, nitrites, and *N*-nitroso compounds (No. 5, 1978)
Nitrobenzene (No. 230, 2003)
Nitrogen oxides (No. 4, 1977, 1st edition), (No. 188, 1997, 2nd edition)
2-Nitropropane (No. 138, 1992)
Nitro- and nitro-oxy-polycyclic aromatic hydrocarbons, selected (No. 229, 2003)
Noise (No. 12, 1980)
Organophosphorus insecticides: a general introduction (No. 63, 1986)
Palladium (No. 226, 2001)
Paraquat and diquat (No. 39, 1984)
Pentachlorophenol (No. 71, 1987)
Permethrin (No. 94, 1990)
Pesticide residues in food, principles for the toxicological assessment of (No. 104, 1990)
Petroleum products, selected (No. 20, 1982)
Phenol (No. 161, 1994)
d-Phenothrin (No. 96, 1990)
Phosgene (No. 193, 1997)
Phosphine and selected metal phosphides (No. 73, 1988)
Photochemical oxidants (No. 7, 1978)
Platinum (No. 125, 1991)
Polybrominated biphenyls (No. 152, 1994)
Polybrominated dibenzo-*p*-dioxins and dibenzofurans (No. 205, 1998)
Polychlorinated biphenyls and terphenyls (No.2, 1976, 1st edition), (No. 140, 1992, 2nd edition)
Polychlorinated dibenzo-*p*-dioxins and dibenzofurans (No. 88, 1989)
Polycyclic aromatic hydrocarbons, selected non-heterocyclic (No. 202, 1998)
Progeny, principles for evaluating health risks to associated with exposure to chemicals during pregnancy (No. 30, 1984)
1-Propanol (No. 102, 1990)
2-Propanol (No. 103, 1990)
Propachlor (No. 147, 1993)
Propylene oxide (No. 56, 1985)
Pyrrolizidine alkaloids (No. 80, 1988)
Quintozene (No. 41, 1984)
Quality management for chemical safety testing (No. 141, 1992)
Radiofrequency and microwaves (No. 16, 1981)
Radionuclides, selected (No. 25, 1983)
Reproduction, principles for evaluating health risks to associated with exposure to chemicals (No. 225, 2001)
Resmethrins (No. 92, 1989)
Synthetic organic fibres, selected (No. 151, 1993)
Static fields (No. 232, 2006)
Selenium (No. 58, 1986)
Styrene (No. 26, 1983)
Sulfur oxides and suspended particulate matter (No. 8, 1979)
Tecnazene (No. 42, 1984)
Tetrabromobisphenol A and derivatives (No. 172, 1995)
Tetrachloroethylene(No. 31, 1984)
Tetradifon (No. 67, 1986)
Tetramethrin (No. 98, 1990)
Thallium (No. 182, 1996)
Thiocarbamate pesticides: a general introduction (No. 76, 1988)
Tin and organotin compounds (No. 15, 1980)
Titanium (No. 24, 1982)
Tobacco use and exposure to other agents (No. 211, 1999)
Toluene (No. 52, 1986)
Toluene diisocyanates (No. 75, 1987)
Toxicity of chemicals (Part 1), principles and methods for evaluating the (No. 6, 1978)
Toxicokinetic studies, principles of (No. 57, 1986)
Transgenic animal mutagenicity assays (No. 233, 2006)
Tributyl phosphate (No. 112,1991)
Tributyltin compounds (No. 116, 1990)
Trichlorfon (No. 132, 1992)
1,1,1-Trichloroethane (No. 136, 1992)
Trichloroethylene (No. 50, 1985)
Tricresyl phosphate (No. 110, 1990)
Triphenyl phosphate (No. 111, 1991)
Tris- and bis(2,3-dibromopropyl) phosphate (No. 173, 1995)
Ultrasound (No. 22, 1982)
Ultraviolet radiation (No. 14, 1979, 1st edition), (No. 160, 1994, 2nd edition)
Vanadium (No. 81, 1988)
Vinyl chloride (No. 215, 1999)
Vinylidene chloride (No. 100, 1990)
White spirit (No. 187, 1996)
Xylenes (No. 190, 1997)
Zinc (No. 221, 2001)

THE CONCISE INTERNATIONAL CHEMICAL ASSESSMENT DOCUMENT SERIES

CICADS are IPCS risk assessment documents that provide concise but critical summaries of the relevant scientific information concerning the potential effects of chemicals upon human health and/or the environment.

Acrolein (No. 43, 2002)
Acrylonitrile (No. 39, 2002)
2-Alkoxyethanols, selected (No. 67, 2010)
Arsine: Human health aspects (No. 47, 2002)
Asphalt (bitumen) (No. 59, 2004)
Azodicarbonamide (No. 16, 1999)
Barium and barium compounds (No. 33, 2001)
Benzoic acid and sodium benzoate (No. 26, 2000)
Benzyl butyl phthalate (No. 17, 1999)
Beryllium and beryllium compounds (No. 32, 2001)
Biphenyl (No. 6, 1999)
Bromoethane (No. 42, 2002)
1,3-Butadiene: Human health aspects (No. 30, 2001)
2-Butenal (No. 74, 2008)
2-Butoxyethanol (No. 10, 1998)
Butyl acetates (No. 64, 2005)
Carbon disulfide (No. 46, 2002)
Chloral hydrate (No. 25, 2000)
Chlorinated naphthalenes (No. 34, 2001)
Chlorine dioxide (No. 37, 2001)
4-Chloroaniline (No. 48, 2003)
Chlorobenzenes other than hexachlorobenzene: environmental aspects (No. 60, 2004)
Chloroform (No. 58, 2004)
Coal tar creosote (No. 62, 2004)
Cobalt and inorganic cobalt compounds (No. 69, 2006)
Crystalline silica, quartz (No. 24, 2000)
Cumene (No. 18, 1999)
Cyclic acid anhydrides: human health aspects (No. 75, 2009)
1,2-Diaminoethane (No. 15, 1999)
3,3′-Dichlorobenzidine (No. 2, 1998)
1,2-Dichloroethane (No. 1, 1998)
1,1-Dichloroethene (Vinylidene chloride) (No. 51, 2003)
2,2-Dichloro-1,1,1-trifluoroethane (HCFC-123) (No. 23, 2000)
Diethylene glycol dimethyl ether (No. 41, 2002)
Diethyl phthalate (No. 52, 2003)
N,N-Dimethylformamide (No. 31, 2001)
Diphenylmethane diisocyanate (MDI) (No. 27, 2000)
Elemental mercury and inorganic mercury compounds: human health aspects (No. 50, 2003)
Ethylenediamine (No. 15, 1999)
Ethylene glycol: environmental aspects (No. 22, 2000)
Ethylene glycol: human health aspects (No. 45, 2002)
Ethylene oxide (No. 54, 2003)
Formaldehyde (No. 40, 2002)
2-Furaldehyde (No. 21, 2000)
Glyoxal (No. 57, 2004)
HCFC-123 (No. 23, 2000)
Heptachlor (No. 70, 2006)
Hydrogen cyanide and cyanides: human health aspects (No. 61, 2004)
Hydrogen sulfide: human health aspects (No. 53, 2003)
Inorganic chromium(III) compounds (No. 76, 2009)
Inorganic chromium(VI) compounds (No. 78, 2013)
Iodine and inorganic iodides: human health aspects (No. 72, 2009)
Limonene (No. 5, 1998)
Manganese and its compounds (No. 12, 1999)
Manganese and its compounds: environmental aspects (No. 63, 2004)
Methyl and ethyl cyanoacrylates (No. 36, 2001)
Methyl chloride (No. 28, 2000)
Methyl methacrylate (No. 4, 1998)
N-Methyl-2-pyrrolidone (No. 35, 2001)
Mono- and disubstituted methyltin, butyltin, and octyltin compounds (No. 73, 2006)
Mononitrophenols (No. 20, 2000)
N-Nitrosodimethylamine (No. 38, 2002)
Phenylhydrazine (No. 19, 2000)
N-Phenyl-1-naphthylamine (No. 9, 1998)
Polychlorinated biphenyls: human health aspects (No. 55, 2003)
Resorcinol (No. 71, 2006)
Silver and silver compounds: environmental aspects (No. 44, 2002)
Strontium and strontium compounds (No. 77, 2010)